the
skin nerd
PHILOSOPHY

Jennifer Rock is the CEO and founder of The Skin Nerd®, including Skingredients®, the Nerd Network online skin community and the Cleanse Off Mitt™, and a multi-award-winning dermal facialist and skin tutor. She is also the author of number one bestselling book *The Skin Nerd: Your Straight-Talking Guide to Feeding, Protecting & Respecting Your Skin.*

With a background in various sectors within beauty therapy, including holistic treatments and training, Jennifer's goal is to spread the word of skin health across the globe utilising technology to do so, with the Nerd Network having been the world's first online skin consultancy and membership service. At present, the Nerd Network is made up of over 15,000 clients from across the planet.

In June 2019, she launched Skingredients, a customisable active, results-driven skincare collection made up of all of the key ingredients that skin needs.

Website: www.theskinnerd.com
Instagram: @theskinnerd
Twitter: @theskinnerd
Facebook: The Skin Nerd

the
skin nerd

PHILOSOPHY

Jennifer Rock

HACHETTE
BOOKS
IRELAND

First published in Ireland in 2020 by
HACHETTE BOOKS IRELAND

1

Cataloguing in Publication Data is available from the British Library

ISBN 9781473680562

Book design and typesetting by Anú Design, Tara

Printed and bound in Italy by L.E.G.O. S.p.A.

Hachette Books Ireland policy is to use papers that are natural, renewable and recyclable
products and made from wood grown in sustainable forests. The logging and manufacturing
processes are expected to conform to the environmental regulations of the country of origin.

Hachette Books Ireland
8 Castlecourt Centre
Castleknock
Dublin 15, Ireland

A division of Hachette UK Ltd
Carmelite House, 50 Victoria Embankment, EC4Y 0DZ

www.hachettebooksireland.ie

Contents

Part 3

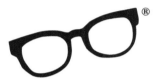

*I dedicate this book to
my mammy, Eilish and my mini me, Matthew.
To Eilish, my mother, a lady with poise,
dignity and elegance. You are a beauty and a creative,
with an admirable attention to fine detail.
My work ethic is unequivocally down to you. You are my rock.
To my Mini Rock, Matthew, who fed me
'feed the skin from within' foods
during the process of writing this book.
You are the absolute love of my life,
my 'why' and my 'why not'.*

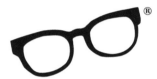

Introduction

Welcome to *The Skin Nerd Philosophy*. I can hardly believe it – a skinquel! With my first book, I remember hoping that some people would discover it, read it and find support and solace in its pages – I never dreamed it would spawn a whole community of like-minded skindividuals and lead to so many joining the wonderful Nerd Network! To this day, I'm blown away by the number of people who have been so enthusiastic, sending me photos of tattered, Post-it-covered book pages on Instagram; the colleges and libraries who have requested to stock the book and use it as a reference guide, not to mention the journalists who still refer to it in newspapers. It makes my soul sing and makes every minute of the hard graft worth it.

Now, following a lot more learning (and the launch of Skingredients), I'm equally excited to bring you *The Skin Nerd Philosophy*. Throughout the book you'll find our foundational Nerdie Principles, which together form the core of the Skin Nerd philosophy – my way of understanding and using skincare. This book is all about a holistic, multi-disciplinary approach to skin health – how you can become an expert on your own skin and skincare, but also how to seek out expertise from others (through research and consultations). My goal is to go below, beyond the skin itself to the principles that guide how we protect, maintain and nourish our skin. The book is broken up into three parts, which focus on:

* What You Need to Consider
* What You Need to Know
* What You Need to Do

In **Part One**, we'll look at the mental aspect of skin and skincare: how we think about ourselves and our skin and why we need to take our skin concerns seriously but not let them rule our lives – a tricky balancing act sometimes.

In **Part Two**, I'll tell you what you need to know to make the optimum decisions for your skin. We will learn by listening to the common questions sent to The Skin Nerd team, by examining some popular – but not necessarily correct – ideas about skincare, and by analysing the typical ingredients found in many skincare products. Warning: it's going to get a bit nerdie in here!

In **Part Three**, we'll get hands-on with skincare routines to suit everyone – no matter how time-pressed you are – and speak to experts such as a dermatologist, plastic surgeon, GP, aesthetic doctor, dietitian and fitness coach among others. You'll nearly have a degree by the time you're done!

We've all had that experience of nervously walking up to a beauty counter, feeling completely unequal to the task of picking out what we need. The rows of gorgeously packaged bottles that scream 'Buy ME!', the assistant who has the mind-boggling spiel ready, the ingredient names that have far too many consonants – tetrahexyldecyl ascorbate, I'm looking at you. It's the Skincare Fear – the feeling that we have no earthly idea what we need, what's in the bottles or how to learn about it. Well, by the end of this book, you won't experience that anymore. You'll be able to stride up to that counter confident that you know your hyaluronic acid from your polyhydroxy acid.

My ambition in this book is to give you the knowledge that makes you feel empowered to make your own best decisions for your skin. Sure, you might need some help to get started – like having an expert consultation with a skin therapist or maybe a chat with your GP – but with education, you can be your own best skin advocate, with the ability to consult the appropriate experts. I want you to feel good in your own skin – to know what is or is not for you, and for you to view skincare as self-care, as a 'me time' investment.

That brings me to what is by far the most important element of the Skin Nerd philosophy, the one you need to take with you as you read, my core belief and goal: skincare must involve a 360° approach. This means that you need to start with the key understanding that the skin is an organ, therefore it must be treated, nourished and maintained from the inside as well as the outside. You are responsible for it, and what you do and the choices you make directly affect it.

In essence, my basic philosophy is that your care for your skin must cover all three fronts – if it's not the full 360°, it's not Nerd levels of skin love and, more importantly, it won't work long-term. It's the holistic approach that sees you in your entirety – skin, body, gut and mind – the whole hooman (a word we at The Skin Nerd use for human!). It is also a jigsaw puzzle, with each piece working in tandem to truly tackle skin concerns and optimise skin health.

Before you dive into *The Skin Nerd Philosophy*, I have a word of advice on *how* to read it. I know you know the bit about following the words and turning the pages – what I'm talking about is how to get the *most* out of it. I've asked so many people about my first book and what they thought of it, and I was struck by how many told me it was brilliant, really informative (thank you, nerds!), but not everyone was sure how to go about making changes.

So this time, I'm initiating the Personal Action Plan in the hope that it will galvanise you into life-changing, unstoppable action. Before you go any further, go old school and get yourself a notebook and pen to keep beside you – heck, write on the book if you want! First things first: write out a list of questions for yourself to really focus on what information will be most relevant to you as you read, such as 'What do I like about my skin?', 'What are my current skin concerns?', 'What would I like to change?', and a list of your own skin questions. A sample list is included at the end of the book.

As you move through the book, write down the answers to your questions as you find them, also noting any advice relevant to your lifestyle. That way you'll have your very own personal guide to what to do next – a tailor-made Personal Action Plan. So instead of turning the last page and (hopefully!) declaring, 'Well, that was helpful', you'll also be saying, 'Now I'm going to take action by taking the steps towards the skin I want to have'.

Your first step might involve a number of things – you might want to audit the skincare products on your shelf, plan out a new morning routine, visit your GP for advice or book a consultation with experts like ourselves. Or perhaps you'll realise that you're already on the right track but introducing some targeted products will refine your routine and make it more effective. Whatever conclusion you arrive at, you'll have the blueprint clutched tight in your mitts. And you can put the notebook to even better use by charting your weekly skin-feel and visual changes, to ensure the actions you've put in place really are delivering for you. Ready?

So read on, and then go forth and be nerdie … change, one skin cell at a time!

Jennifer Rock

1

What You Need to Consider: The Thinking Behind Modern Skincare

It's all about you, you beautiful hooman®!

The key understanding of any skincare routine is this: you are a total and utter skindividual. There are ingredients that all skins can benefit from – and, in my opinion, need – but it's about finding a routine including these that works for you. Yes, you can benefit hugely from professional advice and guidance, but at the same time *you* play an essential role in your skin's health.

It's the old 'with great power comes great responsibility' conundrum. On the one hand, that's a reassuring idea – that you have the ability to nurture your skin and maintain its health. On the other hand, it can feel daunting, especially if you are overwhelmed by the huge volume of skin products available and the amount of information coming at you from all angles – including misinformation and conflicting information. If you have a medical skin condition, the ideal approach is for you to seek expert advice (from a doctor and a skin expert) and follow a tailor-made plan – part of this process might be realising that your power to effect change might be limited and so you will need to work with what's possible.

What I want you to know is that you're not alone in this. The Skin Nerd philosophy is based on the three Es: education, enlightenment and empowerment. In this section, I want to **educate** you about the ways we are encouraged, and discouraged, to think about our skin. I want to **enlighten** you about the importance of healthy skin – what 'healthy' means and how it links into your overall health and wellbeing, including your mental health. And, ultimately, I want you to feel **empowered** to make informed and effective decisions for your skin, body and mind.

The Skin Files

I strongly recommended using a Skin Diary in *The Skin Nerd*, and it's a recommendation I'm going to make again! It sounds like a faff when someone says to write down your feelings and thoughts and how your skin feels to the touch every day, but I really can guarantee that it's worth it. It shows you patterns you likely wouldn't register otherwise, and that is extremely useful skinformation for you to have as the basis for your Personal Action Plan (so you need to add a second notebook to your shopping list now!).

A daily or weekly Skin Diary tracks how your skin feels, if it reacts to anything, and how it behaves depending on how you're behaving. It will soon shed light on what your skin loves and loathes – and you can ramp up on the love!

Here are the headings for your Skin Diary:

* Sleep – how many hours per night
* Screen time – number of hours of blue light exposure

* Daylight – how much time you spent in the sun
* De-stressing – if you had 'me time', and how much
* Water – how much did you consume?
* Sugar – how much did you consume? (can track information on food packaging or just note types of food you eat for your own reference)
* Protein – how much did you consume?
* Carbs – how many carb-rich foods did you consume?
* Good fats – how many did you consume?
* Caffeine – how much? Honestly!
* Alcohol – more honesty! How many units?
* Skincare – what products did you use?

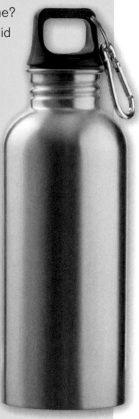

Phew! I know that looks like a lot – it is a lot – but these are the key indicators of skin behaviour and triggers. (We'll discuss diet in more detail on page 41.) And your Skin Diary doesn't need to be a physical notebook – use a notes app on your phone if easier.

Whatever way you think makes sense for you and will be easy to maintain, do that. If you can even do it every day for one week, you'll soon realise that it's worth it and it'll be much easier to keep it up then. You'll be able to track back to find the source of breakouts or redness or dryness or oiliness. It will tell you if your skincare routine is covering all the bases, or if it needs a bit of a rethink. And if you opt for a skincare consultation, your expert will go down on bended knee and thank you for your diligence, because this is the Holy Grail of skinformation!

Maintaining a Skin Diary over a period of a few months will enable you to notice patterns, peaks and troughs so you and/or the expert can alter your regime specific to those (e.g. hormonal fluctuations, work stresses, busy travel schedule) in order to best protect your skin.

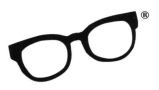

Chapter 1

The Work-(Sk)in-Progress

This is our starting point: I urge you to readjust your thinking and accept that your skin's *health*, as opposed to how it looks, is your first priority and is always a work in progress. Skincare isn't a destination, it's a process, which means you are continually working on your skin health, making improvements, focusing on feeling better in your skin. The work-(sk)in-progress philosophy means that you work hard on your skin with the 360° approach – inside and outside – and your skin will continue to make progress. And sometimes if it doesn't, or if it slides backwards unexpectedly, then you reassess, identify the cause, find the solution and act.

Your job is to make the best choices you can each day, by allocating time for a solid skincare routine, even if it's only a 60-second one (which I'll outline for you later), and investing a bit of time in figuring out what truly works best for you. This won't take too long, but it will be time well spent. Once you're equipped with the knowledge to understand skin products and choose wisely, you're set for a lifetime of skin-specific choices. And once you make a little bit of time in your day for skincare, it will become a habit and you'll come to enjoy and appreciate it. You will feel good in your own skin. And that's a nerdie promise!

The First Nerdie Principle

Our skin is the largest organ of the body and is composed of three key layers: the epidermis, the dermis and the hypodermis. Together they work to protect our insides from everything on the outside, then at night-time they carry out damage repair and generate new cells, which is why sleep is so important for healthy skin. Your skin is an incredible organ, built to be a self-managed system, and yet it is affected by intrinsic factors, such as genes, hormones, the menstrual cycle, gut health and medical circumstances, as well as by extrinsic factors – many of which are within our control, such as sugar intake, tobacco, alcohol, stress and excessive exposure to UVA and UVB rays from the sun. An organ is not immune to anything, which means it needs you to be the sensible filter. Your skin *really* needs *you* to perform this function. You're its minder.

This is why a three-pronged approach to protecting and promoting your skin's health every way you can is so important:

1. **Inside**, by eating nutritious food, taking supplements if necessary and living a healthy lifestyle.

2. **Outside**, by boosting our skin's defence and its efforts through targeted skincare products and professional treatments.

3. **On top**, by protecting the skin with daily SPF and with makeup (if you choose to wear it).

Do You Have Flawless Skin?

Well, straight up, the answer is 'No'. Let's just address the elephant in the room – there is no such thing. I meet people all the time who stare at my face while I'm talking, and not in an absorbed, listening-so-hard-to-you-oh-wise-one kind of way, but in a 'so does Jennifer Rock have perfect skin?' way. That answer is also 'No'. I work really hard on behalf of my skin, but it's not perfect. Some days it's in good condition, some days I have a breakout, some days it's a bit dehydrated, some days it's a bit oily. And I have open pores and – imagine – a wrinkle! Now, I know what to do when any of those things irritates me, but the point is that it still occurs. It can be difficult to accept this fact, but the fact remains: skin doesn't respond to your efforts by reaching a state of perfection and then plateauing there. I wish it did. But it doesn't – and that goes for every single one of us.

The Skin Nerd philosophy is that we should banish the words 'flawed' and 'flawless' from our vocabulary. They are unhelpful words that describe unhelpful notions. If you accept the idea of 'flawless', it means perfect skin is possible and that every skin type that isn't 'flawless' is automatically 'flawed'. It creates a spectrum that has the impossible at one end and natural at the other end; natural should be respected for the wonderful thing it is but instead it can be labelled as 'not perfect', 'not desirable' and 'not damn good enough'. But this is not the internal narration we wish for. In my eyes, we should be working towards skin health and the confidence that comes with it – we are not working towards perfection.

The idea of 'flawless' skin is embedded in beauty culture, which promotes the concept that skin can be perfected. It's common to point the finger at social media for this, with its Photoshopping, filters and enhancing ring lights. However, long before everyone was uploading their filter-perfect pics online, magazines were selling us the idea that some women and men – the ones on and between their covers – had flawless skin and the rest of us had to chase this ideal. (That was at a time when the magic tricks of good lighting and a tweak in Photoshop weren't as commonly understood.) The means of getting that message across have changed, but the message has been the same for a very long time. If you think about it, women in the eighteenth century weren't poring over Insta-stories of girls with white-powdered skin and bouffant hairdos and yet somehow the message of how they 'should' look was transmitted very effectively. It's a social and cultural reality, and it's been there as long as mirrors, practically. We all strive for the next level of beauty, whatever we may perceive that to be, in whichever era.

But if we understand the tricks of the trade – the filters and lights – that are used to achieve the 'flawless' look, you won't have to dwell on the fact that how you look in real life might not be in any way like how people look online. You will know how to separate fact from fiction, perfect from natural, filtered from non-filtered.

Often, celebrity skincare routines are unimaginable – and unattainable – to the normal Nerd. I'll give you an example: I trained a therapist whose fulltime job was treating and maintaining the skin of one celebrity client, keeping it in tip-top condition. This therapist was on-call 24/7 and had access to all of the most advanced skincare technologies and techniques, on demand. The entire focus of her working life was this one woman's face and body, alongside a surgeon, doctor, manicurist and hairstylist. Brownie points for dedication and investment! So yes, people like this client look exquisite in pics, but they can spend any amount of money on their skin and – crucially – can spend lots and lots of time on it, too. Their regime might involve dedicated

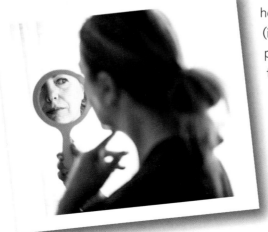

teams of stylists and therapists, two-hour facial peels and multimodality (involving multiple tools) treatments per week, hours with their personal trainer and meals green-lit by a nutritionist and prepared by an expert chef. It's a level that's totally beyond most normal people – so why compare yourself to that and feel pessimistic?

Respect the Skin You're In

The idea of loving your skin, accepting it and respecting it might be a radical one for some people. But our skin is the outward 'self' that greets the world so how we feel about it is incredibly important. We are all only hooman, which means we can sometimes get hung up on negative ideas, particularly ones about ourselves. If you are constantly comparing yourself to others – your friends, siblings, celebs – then you're potentially going to be establishing an unhealthy competitive or perfectionist mindset.

So what does a healthy mindset look like? It all boils down to accepting your skindividual state, embracing it, respecting it, working with it. There is a whole host of circumstances – external and internal – that contribute to creating your skin state. That's why it's not the same as anyone else's. Your skin state is a constant work (sk)in progress and therefore is constantly changing, affected by things both within and beyond your control. This means that the best thing you can do is to focus on healthy skin rather than being driven by aesthetic goals (the same way a focus on diet should be about healthy eating rather than about fitting into a tiny pair of skinny jeans) – meaning the healthiest skin you can achieve given your specific circumstances, genetics, lifestyle and time available to you.

There are many competing definitions of 'healthy skin', but I'd say that healthy skin is skin that has its unique concerns addressed with a bespoke daily care routine, that is protected, treated and nourished according to its specific needs. This means that you consistently – yes, every day, no skiving off – perform the basic skincare tasks of cleansing and applying serum and SPF to optimise your skin's health. As we've said already, try not to focus on the idea of a final goal. It's a work in progress that's ongoing and changing throughout your life and with every season, depending on hormones and lifestyle. There are so many interlinked factors involved that there is no endpoint – as your life changes, your skin changes. Your skin is with you through the ups and downs of your life: it may thrive when you have the time to exercise regularly and eat well, but the hard and stressful times will affect it too.

Promoting Skintegrity

* Respect your skindividual needs – understand that your skin is unique and must be treated as such.
* Knowledge is power – educate yourself so you can make the best choices for your skin.
* The 360° approach is the best way to achieve healthy skin in the short term and long term.
* Accept your skin for what it is, and what it could be – don't be seduced by the idea of 'flawless perfection'. Repeat after me: IT. DOES. NOT. EXIST.

Real-life Skin Journeys

The Nerd Network is our term for the community of people who have joined and become members of the Nerdie world, starting with an online skin consultation with one of our team of expert Nerds and Nerdettes. They are always eager to learn about skincare and trade skinformation with each other, they share their real-life experiences of skin, treatments and products, and we learn a huge amount from them – their desires, requests, concerns … we are constantly listening.

Our focus as experts is on how skin *feels* rather than how it looks. Instead of dwelling on skin issues we ask: Does your skin feel better today than last week? Do you feel happier about your skin? How does this new routine feel to you? Do you feel better without makeup on? We want your skin to feel the best it can, and for you to feel the best you can too.

Feeling good is a very individual thing and a highly relevant one, and we at Nerd HQ believe what is important is how our skin feels right now, not where it is on the spectrum of 'good' to 'bad'. If you're putting in the work, you'll be feeling the improvements. You need to recognise that progress, enjoy it, be proud of the steps you are taking to look after your skin. The best way to do this is through your Personal Action Plan, which will soon reflect back all your hard work in positive entries. We all need recognition of our efforts in order to maintain them, so focus on how your skin feels and keep up the work so that it keeps feeling better and better. It's all about ongoing progress – that's what the Nerd Networkers will tell you.

I wanted to tap into the real-life skin stories of the Nerd Network, so I created a survey to find out what they thought about their skin, and what they felt worked – or didn't work – for their skin.

Our first question on the survey was about people's skin condition before joining the Nerd Network. In the 'before' period, 40 per cent of respondents said that their skin had made them feel insecure, 20 per cent said it had made them feel sad and 45 per cent said they didn't feel confident going without makeup. One respondent said, *'I would go as far as saying I was depressed because my skin was so bad, and I felt like everyone noticed.'* Another said, *'I had been struggling with my skin since I was 14. I felt so ugly and gross and it actually depressed me. I couldn't understand how my boyfriend found me attractive when I looked in the mirror and saw such terrible, horrible skin.'* Comments like this are hard to read, but they reiterate the emotional connection to skin health. It certainly confirmed my long-held belief that how we feel about our skin goes to the very heart of how we feel about ourselves. This is why skincare to me is not vanity but about the physical and psychological effects skin health can have – reading words like 'sad', 'depressed' and 'ugly' is powerful as they make me think, breathe and realise the difference I can make to a person's life. When asked why they joined the Nerd Network, a mahoosive 60 per cent agreed that they wanted to improve their skin health and thought we were the right experts for the job. Hearing people talk about skin health and maintenance of health made my heart thump with joy! When thinking about seeking skin help, 86 per cent said they opted for The Skin Nerd because they knew it was run by experts – this shows that even in the age of skincare self-education, people still respect and want advice from qualified, trained people who can show them the way.

What were your skin concerns when you first joined the Nerd Network?

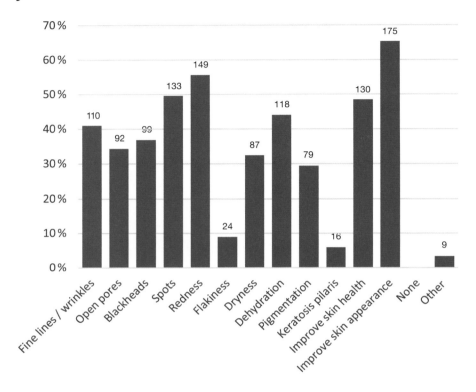

The core skin concern was redness (55 per cent) – no surprise there considering it is a real curse of any Celts with pale skin. Half of the survey respondents said they considered spots a concern, with dehydration coming in just behind at 44 per cent and fine lines and wrinkles at 41 per cent. In the 29–40 per cent bracket, we see concerns like blackheads, open pores, dryness and pigmentation. So it is clear that these are common concerns. At least one of them is probably sounding familiar to you. Totally normal; we all suffer from these issues, but they also can be improved! As for their goals (again, these probably sound familiar): these range from improving skin appearance, improving skin health specifically, and wanting to feel more confident in their skin. That last one makes total sense to me – I think many of us spend our lives trying to build up our confidence and our skin can be a big part of that.

I was curious as to what might put people off seeking help because this is something I often see – people who come to us after a long time living with a skin condition when they don't have to. So we asked, and they answered. The Network confessed that what had prevented them having a consultation with a skin expert was the hassle of trying to find the time to get to a salon or clinic, the idea that facialists can be biased towards recommending the brands they stock alone, and the plain old awkwardness of talking to a stranger about their skin at all. And, of course, being makeup-free can be a vulnerable experience. This might be a feeling you recognise too. But once they successfully pursued seeking a consultation, they were always happy they did so.

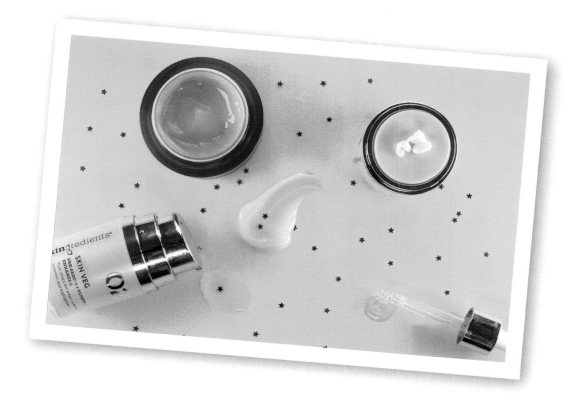

How do you feel about your skin now that you've started following a skincare plan?

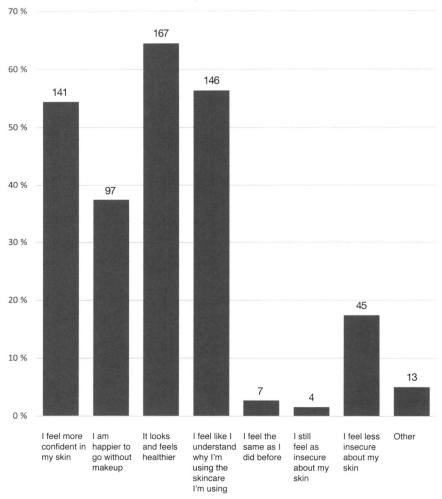

So, now that we've discussed the personal value of skin health, let's ask the big question: what does healthy skin feel like?

Healthy skin:

* feels smooth in the majority of places
* has fewer visible pores

* has reduced/minimal redness
* reflects light
* has a balance of oil or lack of oil
* has minimal pigment
* feels hydrated
* bounces back
* has no impairment to healing ability
* is non-reactive.

And here's a tough question to answer: how long before you can expect your efforts to start delivering that healthy skin feeling?

Well, there's no definitive answer, as you can imagine, although 28 days is the general guideline for skin cell turnover and to see visible differences. But I can break that down a little more and tell you that you can:

* Change hydration levels on Day 1
* Change skin texture on Day 3
* Change skin health, i.e. clarity, pigment, redness, in two to three weeks.

Longer-term benefits, like helping to reduce the appearance of a line, do need at least 28 days.

This is why skin health depends on consistency and effort over time. But (as you can see from the 4 per cent on the graph) it might not happen in a straightforward way unfortunately – hopefully a follow-up consultation or the expertise of a GP or dietitian will help as the next phase of treatment. The best way to see it is as a lifelong choice.

PROTOCOL:
How To Manage Your Skin Expectations

In my career, I have come across a lot of people expecting major results extremely quickly when they start to use new skin products, even though this may not be realistic. A skin expert will be able to tell you what to expect from your new routine, when you can expect to see changes in different skin concerns and when to come back and touch base if you're not seeing results. But it's still good to check in with yourself. Take pictures and try to monitor your skin from a less emotional perspective. Find a skin expert who will be honest, will deliver a skin appraisal professionally and remain focused on achieving the results you wish for, although it may take time and effort. Managing expectations is key in skincare – set small, achievable goals for your skin. For example, pigmentation may have taken 20 years to manifest on your skin, so it will certainly not resolve itself overnight.

Step 1: Take a good, hard look at yourself

Really do. Stand in front of the mirror and take stock of the changes you'd like to see in your skin. Be realistic and focus on small, healthy improvements. Don't get too close, though. People don't usually stand an inch away from your face, and you rarely do it either. Ask yourself:

* How do I feel about my skin's hydration?
* Is the skin tone even?
* Are those 'freckles' darkening in the summer? Could they be pigmentation?
* How much do the blackheads bother me?
* Does my skin heal quickly?

If you want to be truly committed, draw up a small chart for yourself with what you want to work on, in order of priority. Everything must be achievable. Then you can use this for your 'self' check-ins, even between your skin appointments. Make sure to check in with your chart at one-month, three-month and six-month intervals – any more than that could be too detailed and may make you feel pressurised.

Step 2: If you're *really* invested, take regular photos

We love a progress pic and there's nothing like being able to say, 'Wow, I'm seeing a difference.' Take one weekly or monthly, store it in a 'skin health' folder on your phone and then you can easily see the peaks (and, inevitably, troughs) of your journey to skin health. This is helpful in two ways: it'll show what is working, and when other factors may have influenced your skin – stress, tiredness, a weekend of boozing or sugary snacks. I don't recommend taking a daily photo – it's simply too often and can lead to slightly unhealthy patterns and focus.

Step 3: Acknowledge the progress that you're making inside too

Having skin that you believe to be imperfect doesn't make you less intelligent, less funny, less kind or less organised. It's important to find ways to make yourself feel better in your skin, such as following skin-neutral influencers. If you feel that how your skin looks greatly affects your self-worth, maybe consider speaking with a counsellor. There is nothing to be ashamed of by doing this – it's an avenue I've encouraged many to follow.

Step 4: Celebrate your progress

Sometimes, when there have been great improvements, we don't celebrate them because we crave even better results. Stop! Be grateful for every day that you wear less makeup or feel more confident. Thank yourself for minding yourself. Turn your skincare routine into the thing you enjoy. Learn to love the process. Taking care of your skin day in, day out, every A.M. and P.M., is the best way to show it that you care.

Chapter 2

Skin Ideals and Realities

There is a multitude of ideas and theories out there vying for your attention, shouting about the best way to think about your skin health, skincare regime and skincare goals. It can feel like a bit of a pinball experience, ricocheting from one persuasive argument to the next as you try to settle on what makes sense for you. In the past five years, two particular ideas have gained a strong following: the Skin Positive Movement and the Skin Neutrality Movement. These are worth examining to try to identify the optimum mindset with regard to healthy skin – remember, many things skin can start with the brain.

The Skin Positive Movement (SPM)

The power of positive thinking is often discussed, and that's based on a very welcome notion – that we should accept ourselves for exactly who we are and not try to live up to an ideal handed to us by someone else. The skin positive movement was born out of the body positive movement, which called out the exclusive 'skinny is beautiful' mantra that has blighted men and women's lives for decades. The goal was to smash any idea of 'normal' or 'healthy' or 'right' with regard to body shape and agitate for a much broader idea of beauty. The body positive movement has definitely made huge strides in this regard, which is a good thing for everyone everywhere, though there is still some way to go.

From that came the equally compelling idea of being 'skin positive'. It started out online, with some passionate advocates uploading unfiltered images of themselves wearing no makeup. They were immediately called 'brave', to which they replied, 'what's brave about just being me?' The idea was that skin, like bodies, comes in all pigments, types and states of health and that no one should feel they need to hide their skin. You've got a spot? You've got dark circles? No need to be ashamed. High redness on the cheeks? No problem. It's all about being a normal person, which means you're not flawless. The SPM encourages us to give two fingers to any suggestion of not being 'good enough' and to reject any sense of discomfort about our skin.

Over time, certain downsides to the movement became apparent. One of the key issues I noticed was the tendency to criticise people's skin habits or judge those who care about their skin's appearance. The idea of not caring about your skin was pushed further, interpreted to mean you shouldn't work to take care of it. Now, that's never going to be an idea The Skin Nerd can get cosy with. In my world, you are investing in the health of an organ. I've heard it so often socially – people who wouldn't say boo to a smoker over their habit, yet they slag off another person for buying an expensive moisturiser or spending money on treatments. They tease others for their 'extravagances' and make them feel bad about them.

I have a number of thoughts on this aspect of SPM. I firmly believe that you should be comfortable in your own skin just the way it is, but also that your skin is worth investing time and money in and that you shouldn't be judged for looking after it. It's normal and reasonable to want to do the best for your skin so that it looks its best and for you to feel your best. Also, the idea of being 100 per cent positive about your skin all the time, every day, no matter what, might be compelling, but it's not realistic for the vast majority of people. The notion of makeup-free selfies is enough to send some running for the shadows, anxious and worried. I'd never judge anyone for that reaction – if you don't feel confident in your skin, it's incredibly daunting. So while I recognise the warm-hearted hug that SPM offers, and it's great when it works, I don't think it's a whole-package solution – as thought-provoking and as encouraging as it is to see and celebrate others in a real way.

Online content creator and author Melanie Murphy often discusses skincare on her YouTube channel (her video about how she treated her acne has received 1.7m views). Here, she talks about a way of thinking that has helped her make progress on how she felt about her skin:

When the internet was still very young, I had a video about my acne go viral and through that, and all of the messages I received from others with acne from around the world, I realised that it's far more common than uncommon to experience breakouts and that to be ashamed of it was, well, silly … like being ashamed of having naturally brown hair. I finally started allowing loved ones to see me without makeup on and it was an enormous weight lifted off me, as I no longer felt the pressure to hide.

When 'you aren't alone' really sinks in, it's like a tonic. Although I learned with time to view my skin as the organ that it is – something I can actually impact through lifestyle changes and skincare tweaks – I still appreciate it for all that it has taught me about society, expectations of women, self-care, self-acceptance and confidence.

The Skin Neutrality Movement (SNM)

So, what about the newcomer on the block – skin neutrality? This is the next step along the path to self-acceptance from SPM and it argues that skin shouldn't have any role in how we feel about ourselves. Again, it comes from a recognition of how much unhappiness skin issues can create, particularly the very common medical conditions, including eczema, acne and psoriasis. When you have to live with a skin condition every day for life, the constant images of airbrushed and Photoshopped 'perfection' can be a royal pain in the *derrière*, let's be honest. The SNM offers an alternative: don't let your skin define who you are as a person, at all. Don't worry about it, just be you, morning, noon and night. But this is easier said than done – I have lived it too.

This movement encounters the same problems inherent in SPM. From my own work with clients and from the thousands of posts and testimonies of the Nerd Network and Skingredients users, I know this stance simply isn't viable or sustainable. Unfortunately, it's extremely difficult to achieve a carefree attitude to skin for most people and trying to do so can create a mental conflict. It's easy to end up feeling guilty for not being totally okay with how your skin looks and feels, and then even more guilty for any efforts you make to improve it. If you're not neutral, are you then automatically vain? No! This is absolutely not the case in my book – this book! I can see nothing to gain from the idea that if you care about your skin, you're somehow failing. To be neutral about their skin is a hell of a lot to ask of anyone – especially a person with a skin condition that requires and benefits from treatment and targeted effort, and often medical attention. The other difficulty is that you could do all that challenging work of trying to arrive at 'I don't give a damn', only to realise that the world around you is a long, long way behind your thinking. Once again, it can create an inner conflict that ultimately doesn't make you feel good about yourself.

Here's an Idea: Introducing the Skin Active Movement (SAM)

After years of thinking about skin and talking about it with many, many experts and clients, for me this has definitely emerged as the most helpful approach: the Skin Active Movement (SAM). This means actively assessing your skin and its needs, actively accepting your current skin state and actively working to improve it by whatever means best suit your concerns, your own achievable goals and, not least, your pocket and schedule.

This is all part of my desire to change the language around skin and skincare so there are no longer 'good' days and 'bad' days or 'good' skin and 'bad' skin. These ideas put pressure on people, so I want to call a halt to them. You need to think only of the best and healthiest version of yourself at any given time, taking all factors – extrinsic and intrinsic – into consideration. Read all about them in Book 1 (I jest!). It means achieving what's really possible, not chasing a fantasy. The BS-free truth is that for various reasons, including good old genetics, which bow to no product, theory or fervent wish, your skin can achieve a certain point of healthiness, its own 'best' (one that will be different from other people's) and you have to accept that. This is your key challenge: active acceptance. But this is the important part: acceptance doesn't mean kicking back on the sofa surrounded by chocolate wrappers, declaring yourself immune to improvement so, hey, I'll just indulge every tasty whim that comes my way … although wouldn't that be simply divine?! (Sidebar: dark chocolate is rich in powerful antioxidants!) I'm afraid that's not going to cut it here either. Acceptance means loving your hard-working skin every day but also turning up for your skin and working every day to help it achieve its optimum level. That's it, Nerdies, true skin love.

There's that thing people say sometimes about someone, and always with quiet admiration: 'they're comfortable in their own skin'. It means someone who is at ease with themselves, doesn't judge themselves or others harshly, physically or otherwise, forgives themselves for their imperfections and feels good about their wonderful bits as often as they can. It's someone who picks themselves up when they have fallen off this thought process and mindset. Comfort is an undervalued word most of the time, but it shines in that idea: comfortable in your skin. One way or another, we all aspire to that.

And that's exactly what the Skin Active Movement wants to help you reach – that point of self-acceptance where you're comfortable with your skin, but also comfortable with working to improve it.

The Second Nerdie Principle

Actively Working, Actively Accepting

The SAM means realistically assessing your skin's health and its healthiest version. That version is entirely unique to you and there's no point comparing it with anyone else's skin or wishing it away. You have to take all of your skin circumstances into account, then identify the best skincare ingredients and regime that fit you and your lifestyle. You demand the best version of yourself and work towards it because you deserve that. But you don't berate yourself for imperfections because that's pointless and makes you feel negative about yourself. While you actively work to improve your skin health in a holistic way, you actively accept where your skin is at today.

One of the recurring problems I see with making skincare a priority is the perception that it is an expensive investment. A lot of people feel uneasy about spending money on skincare, either because they can't afford it, or see it as unnecessary, disliking the connotations of it as a luxury indulgence. Or maybe they simply can't afford to spend much on it – as a result, many people just won't go there. But it doesn't require excessive spending to make healthy choices. I think a huge stumbling block is the misconception that expensive is superior. It's easy to fall into the trap of thinking you're making the very best, very healthiest choice if you shell out a wodge of cash for a product – like it's a guaranteed elixir. But that is not necessarily true. That's why it's so important that you equip yourself with the tools to be able to assess what products are offering beyond their sales pitch, so you can weigh up the pros and cons. Look

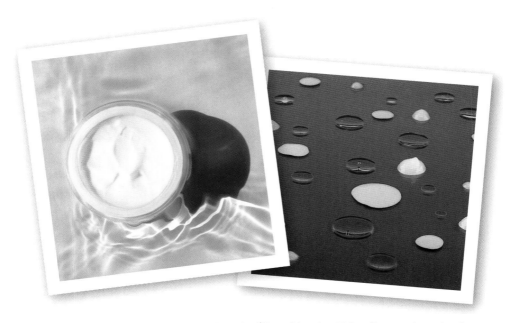

for the data, statistics and clinical trials. (See Chapter 5 for tips on how to do this research.) Nerd it out!

I really learned this while formulating the Skingredients range, which is designed to be results-driven yet accessible. If your skincare budget is tight, this doesn't mean there aren't lots of options available to you to help achieve optimum skin health. It's important that the products you buy are ones that can be used every day rather than ones you feel you need to save for as a once-in-a-while treat.

PROTOCOL:

The Key Rules of the Skin Active Movement

- I'm saying this again: don't judge your skin by how it looks in an extreme close-up in the mirror. That's just not fair on yourself. Go by how your skin feels – hydrated? soft? – and think about what you want to address.

- Remember that you have some control, but you don't have total control, so give yourself a break if you're putting in the effort. Nutrition experts often quote the 80/20 rule: make healthy choices 80 per cent of the time and don't beat yourself up for the less wonderful 20 per cent. That's a good way to look at skin as well – you deserve good choices, you'll enjoy the results but you're only human, so don't try to control-freak it because it won't work. Life happens, hormones happen, we all know that! But keep in mind also that there are ways to impact the fluctuating skin responses with diet, stress management and topical skincare.
- Recognise that the skin is an organ and requires ongoing effort – and frankly, it deserves it too because it's incredibly hard-working and too often taken for granted.
- Remind yourself that medical skin concerns are just that: medical skin concerns – you wouldn't judge a person for having IBS or any another illness they can't control, so treat yourself with that same respect and empathy. Learn about your skin, monitor flare-ups so you can hunt down the causes, then draw up a skincare plan that will work with what your skin needs. And if you need medical attention, seek it out. Bear in mind, skincare can also work to help the outside while the inside is being tackled. (We'll look at the brain–skin connection in Chapter 3 and how it affects common skin conditions.)

Chapter 3

A Skin State of Mind

There has been a fascinating and very important development in our understanding of skin over the past ten years, thanks to the growing influence of psychodermatology. This is a recognised field which draws on the expertise of psychologists, psychiatrists and dermatologists and uses that cross-discipline insight to examine the causes and consequences of skin conditions and skin disease. It's been gaining ground since the 1990s and is now rightly viewed as an essential consideration for those who need ongoing dermatological care. Psychodermatology recognises that skin and mental health can often be very closely linked. If you have a condition that you live with, it's highly likely that it's affecting your brain/mood and that your brain/mood is affecting it, so you really need to know how this works.

Psychodermatology is a science, based on neurology, dermatology, the central nervous system (CNS) and the functions of the immune and endocrine systems, which are all involved in the interplay between brain and skin. Let's look at it in more detail.

1. There is a brain–skin connection

Skin forms part of the peripheral nervous system, which connects with and talks to the central nervous system. The skin is responsible for mediating information relating to touch, temperature, pressure and pain, all part of its main job of forming a protective barrier between the outside world and our sub-skin bodies. The skin and the brain interact and what happens with one can impact the other and vice versa. This might all sound very obvious, but it took decades of research before this skin/brain link was fully established and accepted. And it tells us that mood/emotion, hormonal levels and psychological factors can all have an impact on our skin health and on skin conditions.

2. There is a central nervous system–skin connection

The central nervous system plays an important role in the brain–skin connection – it operates as a messenger between the brain and the skin. This is important because the central nervous system forms part of our immunity defences. In some skin disorders, the system of interrelations between the nervous system, immunity and our skin can become destabilised, and can lead to inflammation, which in turn can exacerbate existing skin conditions. Essentially, a very vicious cycle. This tells us that some skin conditions, such as acne, eczema and psoriasis, can be caused or further exacerbated by the inner workings of the nervous system and are not necessarily caused by the actions or inactions of the person who must live with them. There is much a person diagnosed with such conditions can do to target and improve them, but there was nothing they could have done to prevent them arising – that was beyond their control.

3. There is a gut–skin connection

A lot of attention has been given already to the brain–gut axis, but more recent research in this area shows that there is evidence to support the long-held view that diet plays an important part in healthy skin, and our gut health is believed to potentially exacerbate specific conditions.

The gut is absolutely teeming with bacteria, some classified as 'good', some classified as 'bad', and the balancing act that goes on in there affects the entire body. The gut bacteria, known collectively as the microbiome, work together to protect our intestines, keep toxins out, muscle in on bad bacteria, halt inflammation and assist in the absorption of the good nutrients in our food. If they aren't happy, we're not happy and it shows outwardly on our skin. One of the side-effects of imbalance is gut inflammation, and every Nerd knows that inflammation always spells not so positive news for the skin. For example, various studies have found disrupted gut flora in patients with acne and seborrhoeic dermatitis (ongoing red, scaly, itchy patches believed to be related to the amount of Malassezia yeast that exists on your skin). And bacterial overgrowth in the stomach occurs in people with rosacea more than it does in the non-afflicted population. So this direct pathway from gut to skin often means that a skin condition is an indication of chronic internal health issues. Remember: the skin is an organ, so it's affected by our gut health just like all the other organs.

4. There is an emotion–skin connection

Psychodermatology also seeks to prove the effect of psychological factors on the skin. Think about it – when you're embarrassed, you blush; when you're intimidated by the idea of, say, delivering a speech in public, you sweat; when you're anxious, you might get itchy. We've all been there! So those are some of the obvious ways in which our emotions can manifest physically on our skin. But this can go deeper. Serotonin, a neurotransmitter, is produced in the gut and therefore is intimately linked to gut health. Serotonin is also closely acquainted with your emotional health because it is regarded as the regulator of mood and emotion. If it's off-kilter, it can lead to depression and anxiety. And what can depression and anxiety lead to? Yes, poor skin health. The healthier you are, in your mind and your body, the healthier your skin. So you can see the bigger picture here: your body's systems – inside and outside – are interlinked, interconnected and interfacing all the time.

Stressed-out Skin

One of the key concerns of psychodermatology is stress. Stress is so important when it comes to skin health that 'How would you rate your stress levels?' has been a question on our Nerd Network consultation form from the very beginning. Stress is at the base of many of the studies and discussions because stress, particularly chronic stress, can have a huge impact on our bodies and our skin, exacerbating the symptoms of skin conditions such as eczema, psoriasis and rosacea. This has now been scientifically proven by the raft of new studies designed to explore this cause–consequence pathway. So, what does stress do within your body? It fires off high levels of cortisol and norepinephrine, the 'flight' stress hormones, which in turn ups the levels of testosterone and/ or oestrogen. When this happens, it leads to inflammation, which physically often means redness and swelling. When there is chronic stress, which means ongoing, continuous high levels of the stress hormones firing off, you get chronic inflammation, which means there is little chance for the body to heal. It's a chain reaction, because this in turn leads to a decrease in antioxidant protection. Antioxidants inhibit oxidisation in the body, a chemical reaction that can damage our cells and go on to impair skin function and processes. The inflammation can also cause a breakdown of collagen and elastin (our skin's structural proteins), which compromises healing and protection. All of this affects general skin health, but really exacerbates medical skin conditions and causes accelerated skin ageing (and keeps on doing so). It's like your very own skin demon perched on your shoulder, causing permanent havoc.

Stress, the exacerbator

The traditional view in dermatology was that stress preyed on the skin and caused eruptions, flare-ups and various ongoing conditions. Now, however, we know that the skin participates in the stress response. Yep, your very own skin actually works against you! When the stress reaction kicks off, your skin isn't just sitting there, weeping in a corner, begging to be left alone. It leaps into the fray, engaging in panicked, hostile communications with the nervous system, the brain and the skin's cells. Chief among

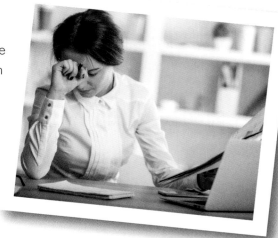

these in the culprit stakes are mast cells – cells that have a role in allergic reactions and parasitic infections – which are located in the nerve endings and blood vessels of the skin and are therefore the first line of defence for the immune system. The problem is, when stress strides into view, the mast cells collude in their own demise by rushing to release stress hormones and inflammatory factors as a means of defence from what the body has perceived as a threat. This is why mast cells are considered to be a factor in many skin conditions, such as psoriasis, atopic dermatitis, and acne. Conditions such as these, and also contact dermatitis, are described as neuroinflammatory, which means they start with inflammation of the nervous tissue. Stress can be the root cause of this inflammation.

As well as compromising the skin's ability to heal effectively, chronic stress can also accelerate skin ageing – the release of cortisol caused by stress can break down the collagen and elastin in the skin causing sagging and wrinkling.

For those of you trying to work with the skin conditions that are exacerbated by stress and inflammation, it isn't the case that it's all out of your hands and there's nothing you can do. Thankfully, there has been and continues to be a huge amount of work on the treatment of conditions such as acne, psoriasis, eczema and rosacea. These tend to receive particular attention because they are so widespread throughout the world, and in Ireland specifically – especially among those with pale skin: fair, freckled and easily sunburned. When working towards optimal health with an ongoing skin condition, you'll need patience and perseverance in equal measure. The first step is a trip to your GP, because these skin conditions require extra care and expert help.

Stressed about our skin

The consequences of skin condition-induced stress can be a really tough subject because it is incredibly personal and involves some of the most difficult emotions we may have to face in life. But it's very important to acknowledge those feelings in order to work on them and hopefully address them, and equally important that those not experiencing such conditions or such feelings gain an insight into them so that they are more understanding of and empathetic towards those who do.

When it comes to the stress induced by medical skin conditions, the emotions can range from shame, to poor self-image, low self-esteem, poor self-confidence, anxiety, depression and even suicidal thoughts. It can be a debilitating experience that steals a person's sense of self and any sense of comfort with that self. It is extremely serious and deserves to be treated as such.

This type of constant stress reaction hugely impacts a person's quality of life (QOL). This is where the brain–skin link is at its most visceral. Those emotions spiralling off from the lived experience of a skin condition have a heavy psychological impact. This is difficult enough as an adult, but can be worse when a skin condition occurs in adolescence, at a time when young people are already self-conscious and often anxious about how they fit into the norm. One of the consequences for people of all ages can be social exclusion, because the person basically doesn't want to go out and be seen, and that brings with it loneliness, which is another really difficult and high-impact emotional state. And, of course, it's a nasty cycle because the resulting stress lowers QOL, the stress of that affects the skin, the skin gets worse, QOL drops further … and on the cycle goes.

Emotions don't stay in their box either – they break out into all areas of life. So when stress has caused this sort of emotional reaction, it can go on to affect relationships, your sex life, your work life, ambition and basically every facet of life that requires you to hold your head up high and engage with people.

I'm not always hugely pro-internet but this is actually one area where it can help: online skin communities show those suffering in silence that they are not alone but one of many, which can be a huge comfort, as noted by Melanie Murphy earlier in the chapter. The power of shared experiences can be life changing, so the online world does have a role to play in helping to tackle and manage stress. It is indeed a community, one in which you can be a spectator or a participant; regardless, it can provide a sense of belonging.

AN EXPERT'S VIEW

Dr Alia Ahmed is a psychodermatologist and a pioneer of this relatively new field of thought. Her first-hand experience is insightful:

People with skin conditions are at a higher risk of developing poor psychological health, meaning they are more likely to feel embarrassed, low, anxious, have body image issues or feel socially isolated. These feelings can then impact their skin and it can turn into a vicious cycle. I would encourage anyone with a skin problem that is affecting their quality of life, or stopping them from doing the things they want, to seek advice from a healthcare professional to see if they would benefit from a psychodermatological approach.

We'll hear more from Dr Ahmed on page 203.

Case study: Concerns

Gary is in his forties and has worked in manual-labour-intensive employment throughout his career.

'I had rosacea and it was very flaky – I'd call it a heated red – and it was sometimes painful. It was a burning sensation, like a tingling feeling that just kept burning on my face. It was only when I was in warm rooms, or if I was after having spicy food. I was completely embarrassed about it. On three separate occasions, I walked into the pub and people turned around and said, "Jesus Christ, what have you

done, what have you been eating, your face is absolutely red raw?" and I ordered a pint, skulled it and turned around and walked out.'

Aoife is in her late twenties and has struggled with acne throughout her life.

'I've had acne since I was 15 years old — mild, moderate and severe — and it has informed more of my decisions than I'd like to admit. My skin has been the thing that I've been most self-conscious about since my teenage years. It has made me angry, sad, hopeless and filled with self-revulsion. It has made me agonise about leaving the house, made me fearful of showing a romantic partner my face sans paint, and very nearly made me turn down a job.'

The Third Nerdie Principle

Understand the link between skin and mental health

There can be a tendency to dismiss skin worries as vanity, or as temporary little niggling anxieties that will disappear. The work of psychodermatology has shown that this isn't the case — these feelings are serious and must be taken seriously. Stress can have a negative effect on our skin. And intermittent or ongoing skin conditions — which, remember, are very common and affect a large percentage of people — cause very real stress, which in turn can lead to further inflammation and flare-ups. Stress can be debilitating and dealing with a very public set of symptoms makes it incredibly difficult. The key thing to accept is that you're not alone, that there is a variety of possible solutions available to you and that you must respect your own feelings and seek the help you need to overcome your particular skin concerns.

What can you do to treat the consequences of stress?

Skincare

A consistent skincare routine is an important ally in breaking the cycle of stress – flare-up – more stress. There are two benefits: first, the application of recommended products will have a positive effect on your skin. Everyone needs to cleanse and hydrate their skin, feed it with vitamins and protect it with SPF – those are the basics.

Secondly, it is recognised by mental health experts that daily routines can help to alleviate the symptoms of anxiety and stress – structure and stability provide familiarity. A good system of self-care should involve a support system/community, regular exercise, a daily routine and avoiding unhealthy behaviours. Your skincare regime can't answer all of these needs, but it can definitely be part of your grounding daily routines that provide the comfort of repetition and reassure you that you are working towards health and wellness. Giving yourself reliable 'me time' in your day can be hugely beneficial – it's focusing, promotes good living and gives you a sense of care and wellbeing – it's you keeping a promise to yourself. The soothing, repetitive motions of applying cleanser, serum, moisturiser and SPF, and feeling the textures seep in and begin to benefit your skin, the sanctuary of a quiet bedroom or bathroom – all of this gives you a little mental boost and provides some respite from the constant busy demands of a normal day. So next time someone is shouting at you for hogging the bathroom, take a deep breath, relax, tell them you're under Nerd's orders and to quit their yammering.

Case study: Actions & Results

Gary: 'Since I started supplements and skincare, I don't know how many people have commented that it looks better, I'm told there's a glow and I feel 100% more confident. The whole flakiness is gone. Some people noticed, some didn't, some ignored it, but I always knew that it was there.

It's amazing how when you're educated about skincare, and I only briefly, how much of a difference it makes.

My skin feels more hydrated especially, it seems to be more balanced. It feels 100% better than what it was. It would have been rough and tight before. If I rubbed my forehead, I'd be looking to see what would have come off on my hand. Now I don't have this problem anymore. I've been told I look younger now! I don't know how true that is, but I've been told I look younger.'

Aoife: 'I currently feel the best about my skin that I have in over twelve years, and that's as a direct result of extremely diligent skincare, following expert advice to the letter, and, of course, heavy-duty prescribed drugs! As it turns out, becoming more educated in my skin has rid me of that helpless feeling – knowledge truly is power.

These days, I am more confident in my skin than ever, and the impact it has on my day-to-day happiness is astounding. It's almost disproportionate. I think I might always be someone who wakes up and has to check the mirror feverishly to see if there are any new breakouts; someone who looks asquint if a partner calls them pretty without any makeup on (à la Katy Perry), but I'm starting to finally feel like my skin and I are on the same team. At 27, it's probably about time.'

Diet

Another extremely helpful way of managing stress is to take a long, hard look at your diet and what it's doing for all those hard-working bacteria in your gut. Now, this has to be a long, hard, *honest* look. Do you tend to reach for the convenient, the quick, the instant sugar hit? If you're consuming a lot of sugary foods, caffeine, alcohol, processed foods and takeaways, it's going to tell in your gut just as much as on your skin. As we now know, the gut and the skin link to the brain, which means your whole mood and outlook are affected too. Believe me, I know it can be difficult to pass up the seductive embrace of chocolate and all the other tempting treats, but it *will* affect your skin and stress levels, encouraging that horrible vicious circle that keeps you in the clutches of inflammation and flare-ups. This is where your Skin Diary can be really helpful: note down what you're eating each day and how your skin feels each day, and then see if you can spot any patterns. You might just need your own personal scientific survey to give you the motivation and insight to improve your eating habits. Your Skin Diary will soon show you that interplay between your brain, gut and skin. (See page 7 for a reminder of what to note in your Skin Diary.)

How to Eat for Skin Health

Eating well ticks all the boxes of providing nutrients for your skin, gut and mind. I am not a nutrition expert, but from my experience researching this topic and speaking with those in the nutrition field, the following nutrients are believed to be especially beneficial for skin health. For personalised advice, speak to your GP or a nutrition expert – we all have different needs! **Note:** all of this advice is intended for those who are not pregnant. If you are pregnant or breastfeeding, you need to get advice from medical professionals specific to your current physical status.

Antioxidants

These are food superheroes that can help our body to handle environmental stressors. Many foods are antioxidant; generous portions of fruit and veg will deliver a good antioxidant hit. But if you want the queen of antioxidant-

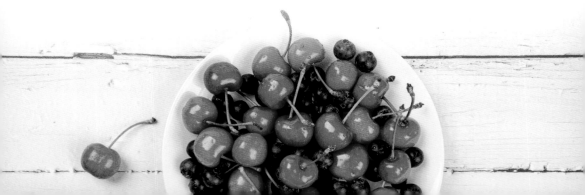

rich foods, you have to indulge in goji berries, smoothies and granola mixes, blueberries and cherries. Hardly a tough ask! Eating a rainbow of foods is usually the key here.

Beta-glucan

This is a bit of a modest super-ingredient as it tends to hide in the shadow of the others and not get shouted about. For me, though, it's a must and I'm always seeking to add it to my diet as regularly as possible. Good sources are mushrooms, oats, barley and algae. You can get algae as a supplement, such as spirulina and chlorella.

B vitamins

There is a whole rake of these, but they fall prey to stress, which depletes them in the body. They do a multitude of wonderful things, so have a look at the table to find out which ones you most need and where you'll get them.

B vitamin type	Food sources
B1 – Thiamin: helps to regenerate collagen, so it's anti-ageing	Wholegrains, beef, pork, eggs, legumes
B2 – Riboflavin: important for effective wound healing	Milk and dairy products, mushrooms, cooked spinach, liver, eggs and tempeh (a soy product). It's also found in cornflakes, so those sneaky cereal 'meals' aren't all bad!
B3 – Niacin: lightening, brightening, hydrating	Portobello mushrooms, potatoes, cereals like bran flakes, porridge, cottage cheese, liver, chicken, turkey, beef, lamb, pork, pumpkin, tempeh and peanuts

B vitamin type	Food sources
B5 – Pantothenic acid: believed to be helpful in reducing acne inflammation	Beef liver, shiitake mushrooms, sunflower seeds and chicken
B6 – good for hormone regulation, so could be helpful if you experience hormonal acne and have flare-ups at specific times in your menstrual cycle	Liver, chickpeas, Atlantic salmon
B7 – Biotin: provides skin's toughness because it's part of the structure of keratin, which is found in hair and nails as well	Meat, egg yolks, salmon, beef liver, sweet potato, sunflower seeds, soy, wheat bran, avocado, spinach
B12 – if you ever get those little white marks on your fingernails, that's your body crying out for some B12. It helps in how the body uses protein, which contributes towards healthy skin cells. A B12 deficiency requires a visit to the GP.	Beef, lamb or veal liver, mussels, oysters

Fibre

Digestion is important for our skin, and fibre is important for our digestion (alongside plenty of water). Fruit such as pears, melon and oranges are rich in fibre, as are peas, beans and pulses. Opt for veggies such as broccoli, carrots and sweetcorn, as well as potatoes with the skins on, and nuts and seeds.

Protein

Our skin has proteins and needs protein – protein fuels our whole body, and thus is integral to our skin. Tofu, tempeh, edamame beans, quinoa, lean meats, poultry and eggs are great sources of protein.

Essential fatty acids (EFAs)

You may be familiar with Omega 6 (linoleic acid) and Omega 3 (alpha-linoleic acid), if only from ads about health food shops. We generally get enough Omega 6 in our diet because it's found in leafy veg, peanuts, grains, seeds, vegetable oils and meat. That's very good news for anyone with sensitivities, sensitisation and inflammatory skin disorders, such as eczema, psoriasis and rosacea, because it helps counteract the underlying inflammation. It's Omega 3 that can be a bit short in supply. For this, you need to deliberately up your intake of salmon, mackerel, mungo and edamame beans, linseed, walnuts, hazelnuts and wheatgerm.

Magnesium

This is important for immune function, and plays a role in reducing acne, promoting healthy barrier function. You can enjoy it in your green leafy veg, like spinach and kale, in fruits like avocados, bananas and raspberries, and in peas, broccoli, cabbage, green beans and sprouts.

Phytonutrients

Your skin will thank you for eating these plant nutrients. Good sources of various phytonutrients include tea, red and white wine (give me an Amen!), apples, peanuts and peanut butter, pistachios, tomatoes, dark leafy greens and egg yolks. But for the best hit of phytonutrients, I highly recommend DIM (diindolylmethane). Don't worry – it's not an exotic veg from some far-flung place – you can find it in the local veg you normally eat – Brussels sprouts, kale, broccoli and cabbage (in other words, the cruciferous family). It's not something you'll hear bandied about much and there aren't any studies I can point to that will scientifically prove its benefits, but I can tell you that I've been using a DIM supplement for years (Advanced Nutrition Programme Accumax supplement) and have personally seen results. I was part of IIAA, the creator of Advanced Nutrition Programme, at the time that Skin Accumax launched, and I saw the trial results, so I have always felt I can vouch for it. I've also seen real results in the clients I've recommended to use it, particularly for acne. I find a delicious way to kickstart the day with a bit of DIM is a kale smoothie.

Probiotics

These are recommended to promote 'good' bacteria and maintain a healthy gut. Personally, I get mine from Udo's Choice, Symprove and ZENii. In terms of food sources, fermented foods like sauerkraut, kimchi, kefir and kombucha are probiotic, as well as natural yoghurt and pickles.

Vitamin A

Our natural stores become depleted through UV exposure, so we need to load up on vitamin A by eating sweet potato, pumpkin, carrots, squash, kale, goat's cheese, apricot and … em … eel – if that does it for you, well and good!

Vitamin C

We don't make vitamin C ourselves, so it's imperative we eat our fill of it. The beauty of vitamin C is its antioxidant properties, which makes it a warrior against mangy free radicals (roving, unstable molecules that damage the cells in your body) and an effective regulator of collagen. So, for plump, younger-looking skin, you need to feast on red and green peppers, kale, strawberries, kiwi, citrus fruits, tomatoes, dark, leafy greens, cauliflower, pineapple, mango, Brussels sprouts and herbs like parsley, thyme and basil.

Vitamin D

This helps fight the effects of age and improves the skin's elasticity and radiance. It also has beneficial anti-inflammatory properties. We normally create our own Vit D through exposure to sunlight, but that can be a hard thing to come by at the best of times, plus our ability to create it lessens as we age. So once you've skidded past 30, it's time to eat it – that means tuna, salmon, eggs, soya milk and fortified plant milks.

Vitamin E

This natural anti-inflammatory and antioxidant armours you against the roving free radicals intent on doing damage. You can eat it in wheatgerm and sunflower oil, almonds, hazelnuts, sunflower seeds, kale, avocado, sweet potatoes and tomatoes.

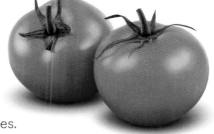

Water

We can't forget about adequate hydration for the skin. The most important thing I'm going to say in relation to water might surprise you: eat your essential fatty acids (EFAs). That might sound odd, but in order to see the benefits of your water intake in your skin, you have to be eating adequate EFAs at the same time. The EFAs help to strengthen your skin's barrier and individual cells, keeping the water in and allowing it to do its thing. So when it comes to healthy skin, water really needs to mean water + EFAs.

Zinc

You don't need very much of this in your body, but even the recommended small amounts will pack a punch when it comes to protecting the fats in the skin, seeing off free radicals and promoting effective healing. There is also evidence to show that it could help in the fight against acne flare-ups. You can get yours in oysters, poultry, red meat, beans, nuts and wholegrains.

When you combine all of the above advice about eating healthily, it might start to look a bit familiar. That's because it largely corresponds to the Mediterranean diet – low on carbs and starches, such as bread and potatoes, but high in oily fish, veg, fruits, beans and nuts. Nutritionists have been recommending this type of diet for a long time, and the dermatologists are happy to give it a thumbs-up, too.

Stress Management

The benefits of a regular skincare routine and healthy eating are clear, but they alone won't solve all of the issues underlying the effects of stress with regard to our skin. Right now, there is no single medical treatment for these inflammatory skin conditions exacerbated by stress. A practical and ongoing approach to managing stress is required. You need to act on the psychological aspect so that your brain and emotions aren't working against you all the time. The key word here is *management*. This is not a curse but a positive – it means the care you choose to give yourself will not be short-lived. It can be difficult to accept this, but accepting it leaves you free to look at the problem realistically and devise realistic responses to it. It's crucial that you become informed about your particular skin condition and arm yourself with the basic knowledge about its known causes, known irritants and known trajectory over the course of a lifetime. This will require you to do some research and maybe have a skin consultation where you can ask all your questions, but it is also hugely helpful to take the initiative yourself and keep up your personal Skin Diary which will allow you to identify patterns, triggers and the factors that make up a 'good day'. This is all crucial knowledge in managing the condition successfully.

PROTOCOL:

Top Three Stress-Management Tips

Bestselling lifestyle author (*Owning It: Your Bullsh*t-Free Guide to Living with Anxiety, The Confidence Kit, NAKED: Ten Truths To Change Your Life*) Caroline Foran shares her top three tried and trusted ways to manage stress effectively.

1. It's not the presence of stress that's the problem, it's your reaction to it

When it comes to managing stress, a lot of us try to do so by avoiding it entirely. We think the key to managing stress is never to feel it, but this is not realistic in the world we live in today, nor was it realistic back in hunter-gatherer times. This idea is also completely counterproductive. Stress is very necessary and important – our stress response keeps us alive. If we didn't have it, we wouldn't last too long. Stress hormones also have some benefits in our lives today in that they can prepare us for something that's important to us - such as giving a presentation at work. Stress also presents itself as a warning that perhaps you're taking too much on or that you need to pay more attention to something that's not serving you very well (such as a toxic relationship). When we try to avoid stress, we wind up just creating more of it. When we resist it, we create friction.

Stress is inevitable and one of the best ways to manage it is to accept it – to a certain extent – as a necessary part of life. Now of course you don't want to find yourself in a situation where permanently stressed out becomes your new normal. That's when you need to look at the lifestyle changes required to bring down that stress response. Stress is something that will pop up and should pop up but ideally it's not going to be the first feeling we greet each morning. When it comes to the occasional waves of stress we're all accustomed to, it's important to remember that it's not so much the presence of stress in your body that's the problem, but rather, how you perceive that stress, or how you respond to it. So accept and expect that stress will come – this alone won't cause you harm; the key lies in what you do next.

Don't try to undo the stress. Don't try to not feel it. Allow for it – this will help it to settle and prevent it from escalating. Try to compassionately understand where the stress is coming from. Look at what's going on in your life. Try to consider what the presence of stress might be trying to tell you and do all of this from a calm, non-judgemental perspective. The worst thing you can do is acknowledge that you're stressed out and then berate yourself for it, creating even more stress hormones in your body. Listen to your stress and allow it to guide you towards the changes you might be able to make in order to prevent 'stressed out' from becoming your everyday experience. What's more, don't feel pressure to justify your stress, or tell yourself you have no reason to be stressed out. It's a physiological response we all have, regardless of our personal situation. There will always be someone worse off than you, but everything you experience is relative to you alone. Telling yourself you have no right to be stressed when life, in general, is pretty good will further enhance the stress you feel, turning it from a helpful nudge into something that negatively impacts your wellbeing.

2. Don't underestimate the power of the breath

Your breath is your anchor, wherever you are, whatever you are doing, whatever time of day it is. It's a tool that's vastly underappreciated but it's one we all have in our arsenal. It doesn't cost a penny either. Whenever you feel stress rising in your body, bring your attention to your breath. Focus on one deep inhale through the nose – allowing your belly to expand with air as the breath goes in – and one slow, controlled exhale out through the mouth. Even doing this once will make a massive difference. By bringing your breath down to your belly and out of your upper chest, you're immediately calming that stress response. Practise deep belly breathing as you do your morning and night-time skincare routine. Practise it as you wait in line for your morning coffee. Get familiar with your breath as a calming tool when you're feeling good so that it's easier to draw upon when you find yourself in a stressful situation.

3. Talk about it

They say a problem shared is a problem halved. When you experience stress and you keep it inside, it can reverberate around your body making you feel worse, with nowhere for the stress to go and no release. Back in hunter-gatherer times, when our fight or flight response was triggered, we would then have the very literal opportunity to either fight or flee the situation. Today we aren't faced with the same physical threats but the stress response plays out in the very same way. In order to provide yourself with a release, it really helps to vocalise your stress. It doesn't have to be dramatic, it can be a simple 'let me tell you about how I'm feeling' conversation with someone you trust. This is what prevents stress molehills from turning into stress mountains. We're often afraid to vocalise our stress response as we worry about being a burden on others, but you can explain to a friend that you just need to put it out there without necessarily needing them to give you a solution to your stress. Just think of it as a release for that fight or flight response. A little door you have the power to open to let the negative energy leave your body. If you don't feel comfortable sharing with a friend or family member, noting your feelings down in a journal is a great way to release stress. If you put it all down on paper you will have addressed and acknowledged it, meaning it will no longer be simmering away under the surface.

Two things that I find very calming in my own routine are deep breathing and facial massage or yoga. The good news is that these two things can quite easily be worked into your daily skincare routine, but it's also beneficial to make some real time for these in your day when possible.

Using Breathing and the Wim Hof Method to Relieve Stress

Níall Ó Murchú is a certified Wim Hof Method instructor, traditional Irish healer and former international athlete (breathewithniall.com). *The Wim Hof Method is a scientifically proven, highly effective way of improving your health, strength and happiness involving a series of very simple breathing exercises, combined with gradual exposure to the cold, and then all of that wrapped up in helping the mind focus a little better.*

The Wim Hof breathing method is simple, but very specific. We take 30 big breaths. Then, on the final breath, we inhale deeply and then exhale. At the end of that exhale, we stop and hold our breath. We hold our breath like this for as long as it is comfortable for us. Then, when we feel like inhaling again, we take a big breath in, hold that inside for 15 seconds and then let it go. That is one round of Wim Hof Method breathing. (You can download a free Wim Hof app that will take you through this.) In this process, as the oxygen levels in the body are going up and CO_2 levels are going down, there are changes that happen to balance hormones and reduce stress. When we're holding the breath, there is a whole series of things that happen that helps the body reset its immune system, balance hormones ... It does a lot, it's simple but the reactions within the body are very complex.

Then we take a part of the breathing, the exhale, and use that in the cold. A cold shower is the most straightforward way of doing this. (Important note: it's advised that we don't hold our breath in cold water, instead focus on trying to breathe calmly)

The technique we use in the cold is the most important one. I'm sure you know how it feels to jump into cold seawater or accidentally turn the shower setting to 'cold' – the body moves to a state of panic. All people have to do in this position is breathe gently in and exhale fully out, and breathe gently in and exhale fully. As these slow breaths start to work, the vagus nerve at the back of the brain is triggered and activates – one of its main roles is to get the body back from the fight or flight state to a place of relaxation and repair. If you breathe in this way five, six, seven times, you'll feel your heart rate drop, you'll feel the body start to relax and the blood pressure going down. This is a very important and very simple technique because when we're under stress, the body reacts in the same way as when we're in the cold. Stress (emotional, physical or chemical) is anything that knocks us out of homeostasis or balance. When this happens, the heart starts pounding, the body releases adrenaline, we go into a state of hyper-vigilance, we're looking for a way to deal with the stress – we want to run, fight or freeze.

When we're stressed our focus becomes very, very narrow, and we can't see the broader circumstances. When we start to breathe in this way, the body will come out of the agitated state and move to a state where it can relax and adapt, then our focus becomes broader again, and we can find a solution and a way to 'escape'. We can take this exhale that we use in the cold and apply it to any stressful situation that we face.

As well as a technique used for reducing stress, it is also one that we can use as a preventative measure. Take two minutes a day – we all have it, set a timer – and breathe like that for the duration. This keeps the nervous system in a state where it can relax and repair and heal. Then, if stress comes, we're in a better position to deal with it and we can tap into that technique more easily as we have the practice.

It's a life-changing tool that you can use at any time. We all face anxiety, fearfulness and worry. Taking control of that exhale means that we can change how we feel and think within a few breaths.

I was an energetic and sometimes difficult child and my granny used to say to my mother, 'If you could just breathe deeply, you could manage him better.' She was nearly right – we used to focus on big breaths in, but it's the big long exhale we want to focus on.

Facial Yoga

Lydia Sasse, @yogawithlydia on Instagram, is a wellness guru, yoga and facial yoga teacher, educator and teacher trainer. Here she gives us some tips on dealing with stress.

If you stop and think about it, when we see a face that inspires us, the thing that usually draws us in is the fact that you can see that person's whole life written there. We can see how much they have smiled, and laughed, and loved. With facial yoga, we can learn to minimise the wrinkles and lines that arrive from sadness and anger, and highlight instead those that come with joy. This is the best kind of self-care – the kind that allows us to hone in on the characteristics that make us feel good and learn to fully inhabit the skin we are in at every stage in our lives. It is not about erasing the character from our faces but instead about celebrating our best bits.

The premise of this type of yoga is that by mastering control over the fine motor skills of our body, we can learn how to begin to unravel tension patterns that we have been holding unconsciously. What this means in practical terms is that we become aware of where we are holding stress in our face and neck, and therefore we can begin to let go of it.

We all know that muscles need to be exercised in order to stay plump and *toned. Facial yoga exercises firm up sagging muscles and help us achieve the youthful glow that we are all after.*

Here are some facial yoga poses:

The Satchmo

Benefits: *tones the muscles of the cheeks.*

Take a large inhale and puff up both cheeks until they are full of air. Then rapidly transfer the air from one cheek to the other for 30 seconds.

The Cheek Pat

Benefits: *boosts circulation and tones the cheeks.*

Take a large inhale and puff up both cheeks until they are full of air. Holding the cheeks to full capacity, rapidly pat each cheek with the palms of your hands for 30 seconds.

The Marilyn

Benefits: *plumps and defines the lips and tones the cheeks.*

Pucker your lips into an exaggerated kiss. Place your index and middle finger on the centre of your lips and then simultaneously push your lips into your fingers and your fingers into your lips, providing resistance. Hold for 30 seconds.

The Forehead Smoother

Benefits: *prevents wrinkles by relaxing the forehead muscles using acupressure to release tension. Can help prevent tension headaches.*

Make a fist with both hands. Place the middle and index finger knuckles in the centre of your forehead and apply firm pressure as you slowly slide your fists out to each side.

End by gently pressing the knuckles against the temples. Repeat four more times.

Part One Skin Takeaways

- The basis of good skin care and healthy skin is Education, Enlightenment, Empowerment. This means you inform yourself, you understand what works for you and what doesn't and this makes you feel mighty – well, it at least makes you feel you know enough to make the right choices for your skin.

- The Skin Nerd approach is to always go by how your skin feels rather than by how it looks because healthy skin is a work in progress. Use your Skin Diary to help you log the effects of your hard work on that skin feeling, learn your triggers and then learn to address them where possible. Seek a consultation; be guided wisely.

- There is no 'flawless' skin on anyone, anywhere – just on Instagram. Every single person on the planet has to feed, water and nurture their skin to achieve and maintain skin healthy status – some more than others, granted. There is no need to demonise yourself if you have breakouts or inflammation or just a dull, tired day. Make good choices as often as you can, and cleanse, moisturise and SPF every day. Be kind to yourself. Be fair to yourself.

- Embrace the Skin Active Movement – actively love it, actively understand it, actively work with it. Live it.

- Eat yourself skin healthy. There are foods that love your skin and foods your skin doesn't love – choose what you eat with that in mind.

- Stress and chronic stress are toxins that affect your body, mind and skin. We can't always avoid it, but we can notice what gives rise to it and how we deal with it. Life is ultimately about being faced with all sorts of situations. But we can try to plan for how to manage them. This is a crucial part of your self-care routine … and your life.

2

What You Need to Know:
The Knowledge to Make
the Best Skincare Choices

Nerdie knowledge is power!

There is a lot to learn and know about skin and skincare. I've spent years getting my Nerd on. Some people look at this as an exciting discovery; some people would rather watch paint dry. If you're the exciting discovery type, then this sweep through the fundamentals that you need to understand will be a thrilling little escapade. If you're already itching in your seat, maybe take comfort from the fact that I'll set it all out very clearly and accessibly and by the end, you'll be glad to have this higher knowledge to call on. I won't apologise for it, though — I am truly a Nerd and I adore the nitty-gritty of skincare.

I often think that skincare is similar to nutrition in that everyone has a rough idea of the right thing to do — they might even scan the ingredients list for 'baddies' — but an underlying sense of defeat can remain. It's easy to think, 'I can't even begin to know the ins and outs of what I need, so why stress over it?' While I understand that feeling, it won't win you any prizes for self-care. That's what a good skincare regime and healthy eating are both about — they are *self*-care. Yes, it might feel like extra things on your already head-melting To Do list, but they are things really worth doing. Let's face it, there are things on that list you could put off for years and it wouldn't have any major consequences: nobody's life has been changed by an underwear drawer clear-out! But when it comes to skincare, you're doing it for the sake of your lifelong health and wellbeing. That's got to trump all the other things vying for your attention. Priorities, people!

That said, you shouldn't feel obliged to swot up on it to the point where you're giving your friends detailed anatomical descriptions of their epidermis. If you want to conduct your own research, we'll explore how to do this in Chapter 5, but if that's not for you, no worries – get an expert in skincare to give you the lowdown on *your* skin and its specific needs. Hey presto, you're an expert on your skin! And that's all the information you really need. You don't have to learn *everything*, you just need to know what you need to know.

It's not difficult to get a good grasp of the basics of skincare. Yes, ongoing scientific developments can update advice, and trends can race in and out and distract you, but at the core of skincare there are essential elements that never change, such as the importance of making the right choices when it comes to your diet and, in topical skincare, the daily holy trinity of **cleanse + serum + SPF**. These are your non-negotiables. Accept them and learn to love them because they are your friends. You don't have to spend huge amounts of money, you don't have to spend hours in the bathroom or on the therapist's table, but what you do need is that reliable basic knowledge, consistency of application of that knowledge and, most

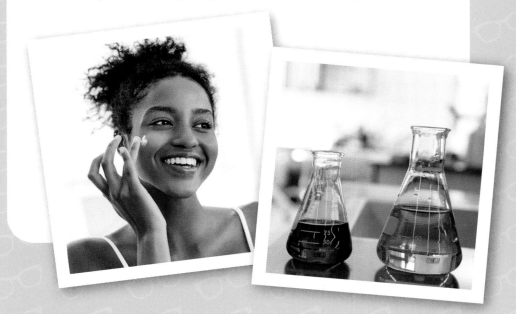

importantly, an understanding that it's what is *inside* your products that ensures they perform their true function. This is Skin Nerd 101: **know what to do and do it, every day, consistently, no quibbling, no slacking off**. The reality is you'll be better off consistently performing a basic routine than doing four different masks but going to bed with your makeup on at the weekend.

In order to give you the knowledge you'll need to make the optimal choices for your skin, we'll start off by looking at the commonly asked questions of the Nerd Network. It provides a great insight into what people do and don't know and what they wish they knew. We'll also look at common misconceptions about skincare, to bust any myths that might be getting in your way and tripping you up. Then we'll examine the whole area of ingredients along with sustainable choices in skincare products because that is a topic of huge and growing interest to so many people. If you want to put your money where your green concerns are, we've got you covered.

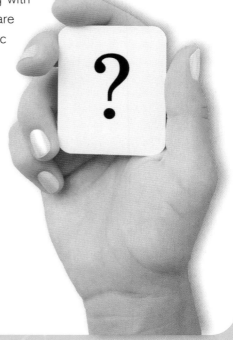

Chapter 4

Your Questions, Answered

Here's an insight into the most commonly asked questions about skincare courtesy of the Nerd Network. Their queries and concerns, which are likely to echo yours, provide a great insight into the gaps in knowledge around skincare. So, I'll pop on my pristine white lab coat for maximum nerdiness, and away we go!

Skin issues

I've got a spot and I need to get rid of it fast. How do I do it?

Probably not the answer you want, but it depends on the type of spot. If it's a small whitehead, dry out the tip overnight with salicylic acid, sulphur or another drying lotion, then tap some hyaluronic acid or antioxidant serum onto it to hydrate it. Sometimes we over-dry it, which leads to pilling and dehydration and slows the healing ability.

If you've been greeted with an angry red spot, although tempting, I can guarantee touching or squeezing it will make it worse. By doing this you can damage the pustule within the pore, spreading the infection and thus inflammation further across and deeper down into the skin. This will make the blemish more noticeable, which will likely make you as angry as your spot.

Again, salicylic acid is your first port of call with a spot of this type. Spot-zap with your strongest salicylic cleanser (preferably 2 per cent salicylic acid) by applying it directly to the spot, leaving it for approximately three minutes, and washing it off thoroughly. If the spot is truly affecting you, gently ice it (with a cloth or a bit of tissue between the ice and your skin) to help temporarily reduce the swelling, but really you just need to be patient and wait for it to go away.

Can I ever pop a spot?

We never answer 'Yes, do it' to this question, but if you're going to, best that it's done properly and only when there is an obvious, white, infected head – never when there are plugs under the skin or a red papule simmering under the surface.

If you want to pop a spot, here is the safest way:

1. Wash hands.

2. Wrap tissue around fingertips.

3. Using the padded tissue, stretch out from spot, downward pressure and wiggle. Stop before there's any blood. Do not place fingers down and at the spot. A sideways angle and a rock 'n' roll motion is better.

4. Place antibacterial solution on the spot once you have popped it because it is now an opening in the skin and is a type of wound. For this reason, I wouldn't recommend makeup directly on top. Leave it to heal properly.

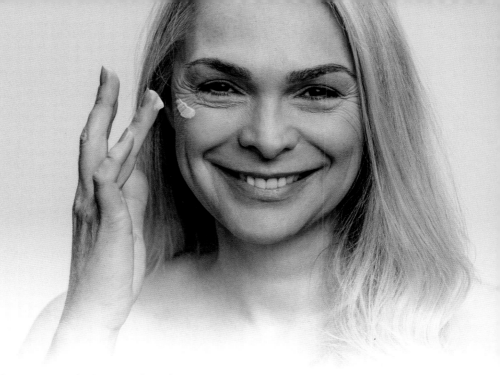

Is there much I can do about wrinkles around my eyes?

Do you want the good news or the not-so-good news? How about the honest news? When wrinkles are already there and in action, there's not a lot you can do that will 'get rid of them' outside of more invasive procedures. However, peptides, vitamin A and vitamin C can improve the appearance of lines and wrinkles, so introduce a serum containing all of them (like Skingredients Skin Protein for your face, neck and eye area or the Environ Skin EssentiA AVST Moisturiser). Always remember to bring your SPF right up around your eyes too because they're definitely not immune to UV damage. If you find that your SPF stings your eyes, perhaps research and consider a mineral SPF as they're less likely to cause a stinging sensation.

Can you make pores smaller?

We can't make genetic pore size smaller. A pore isn't a muscle, it's just an opening in the skin. However, pores can become damaged over time due to spot popping or degradation of collagen and elastin due to lifestyle factors. Remember, from 25 years of age onwards, your skin's natural ageing process is affecting it too. Improving general skin health and upping the collagen your skin is making can improve the appearance of your pores … over time.

For those who need more focused action, microneedling can help to make pores appear smaller by rapidly bringing about the skin's healing cascade which stimulates elastin and collagen production.

Be wary of falling into the common trap of overusing acids like salicylic acid, thinking you're assisting in reducing pore size by keeping pores clear. You may find it is merely that the elastic bounce is less, rather than pores being 'clogged', as is frequently believed. Remember that we are targeting elastin, the protein that helps to give our skin elasticity, and is key to preventing the excessive degradation of pore size as opposed to solely the oil secretions.

I've tried skincare, antibiotics, a dairy-free diet, clinical treatments and acne supplements for my acne but nothing's worked. Is Roaccutane my only option?

Firstly, acne is a medical condition, so whatever is advised and prescribed will be your best route. The options you tried so far can definitely help to improve acne and even reduce the severity when used regularly, but we would recommend an expert skin consultation first – and dairy-free is subject to controversial discussion! Some of us out here in the world could be eating raw food diets, cleansing like champions, having peels as recommended and the like … but at the end of the day, Roaccutane may be the most effective, long-term option (see page 236 for more information). I've been on it myself in the past (and my congestion still flares due to stress, for example).

It is a medication with much opinion surrounding it and can only be recommended through a dermatologist as referred to by your GP. When researching it, keep your health in mind and always be guided by the dermatologist rather than blogs, as it is a medicine.

I have blotchy redness that gets worse when I drink alcohol. Why is that?

I'm afraid it's likely you have the gene that causes the skin to redden when you drink – the flushing is caused when your body makes too much of the enzyme that breaks down alcohol. Unfortunately, there's not a lot you can do about it except to avoid or limit alcohol consumption. Many makeup artists recommend using a yellow-based concealer on the areas that become red if you are planning to have a drink. Vitamin C is key for redness longterm, inside and out. Identify your triggers (could it be caused by over-exfoliation or products stripping the skin barrier?), track in your diary and follow up with your Personal Action Plan.

It's also possible that you have rosacea, a long-term medical skin condition that usually causes blotchy redness, heat and irritation – this should be diagnosed by a doctor. Alcohol is a known rosacea trigger, so drinking may exacerbate the symptoms. If you have these concerns alongside other symptoms, I'd recommend you speak with a medical professional to discuss it further.

My skin looks terrible when I'm hungover. Why is that?

Scenario: you wake up after an evening of fun to a tired, bespotted face in the mirror that doesn't look like you at all. Why? Multiple reasons. Alcohol is a diuretic, which means you pee more and rid yourself of hydration, leading to the physical manifestation that is 'drinkles' – a word we coined to describe wrinkles caused by dehydration. It also destroys your sleep pattern and therefore your skin cannot perform its usual processes as well, which gives you that dull, grey pallor.

Alcohol may affect the systems within us that determine whether we'll get a spot, but for the most part I'm convinced that another reason we're spottier after drinking is because we're not as good at removing our makeup while under the influence. And, of course, that's on top of sugar-filled alcoholic beverages, late nights and perhaps fast food, which will all trigger inflammation alongside the alcohol. Feel free to hone your skills in cleansing while merry by standing on one leg and closing one eye every night.

The best way to avoid looking not as sprightly the next day is to limit your alcohol intake, and many experts recommend following each alcoholic beverage with a glass of water.

Skincare

Should I change my skincare products regularly?

Let's keep this one short and sweet: if it's working for you, nope. No need. So long as you're getting a great combination of nourishing, hydrating, protecting and hard-working ingredients onto your skin, you can stick to the same routine until your skin needs change. If your skincare isn't getting the results you crave anymore, then you can add something in or swap it to up the ante! And to be clear, 'working' doesn't mean 'lack of negative reaction' – we can set the bar a little higher than that. We wish and aim to work towards healthier, brighter, noticeable differences.

All routines can benefit from fine-tuned tweaking – increasing antioxidants at times of stress, or upping ceramide levels when the skin is dehydrated – but in essence the core ingredients (vitamins, peptides, hyaluronic acid, antioxidants, SPF and, if applicable, exfoliating acids) are needed 365, 24-7. These ingredients will be discussed in detail in Chapter 6.

My skin's in good condition but a little bit dry. What can I do to help?

I understand 'good condition' to mean normal pore size, normal oil production, even skin tone, lines and wrinkles that you feel fit the age you are. I'm also assuming you're using a solid skincare routine as outlined in this glorious tome.

If you're fairly healthy on the outside, take a look at the inside. Do you eat enough good fats through your diet or supplements to support your skin's barrier? An omega supplement or, for the plant-based, a flax supplement may be just the thing you need to keep your skin locking in moisture.

Topically, make sure you're getting an abundance of different types of hydrating ingredients through different parts of your routine: humectants (such as hyaluronic acid) draw in moisture, emollients (like shea butter and fatty acids) soften and hydrate the upper layers, and occlusives (like squalane and shea butter) lock in moisture. A lot of products and ingredients are both of the last two types. For example, silicones are usually both emollient and occlusive. If you're genetically dry, it's usually down to you not making enough sebum (oil), so using a facial oil will help too.

I've oily skin and I like using a toner to keep me less oily. What's the harm?

Traditional astringent 'oil control' toners are, for the most part, alcohol-based and work to temporarily reduce oiliness. They do this by dehydrating the surface of the skin, which may lead to more damage over time and will make you instantly look older – a raisin versus a grape, if you recall from my first book. Skip them and opt for something that does the same job but benefits your skin, like a salicylic acid cleanser or the Neostrata Refine Oil Control Gel, for example, which contains mandelic acid (an alpha-hydroxy acid) to help with oil control plus polyhydroxy acid to assist in surface exfoliation. These are 'toning' steps with a purpose. Personally, I opt for treatment toners as opposed to toning for the sake of the step, such as the REN Ready Steady Glow Daily AHA Tonic for exfoliation and brightening, or the Environ Youth EssentiA Vita-Peptide Toner for additional anti-ageing benefits in your routine. So toning with a purpose, i.e. containing active ingredients, is a yes, but toning with cotton pads for the purpose of ritual is a no! Spritzing with a facial spritz or mist is comparable to active toning as it hydrates, acts as an anti-inflammatory, and the skin being somewhat wet prior to serum application can aid penetration.

Is it always a bad thing to stick to one complete range from one brand?

I actively encourage the pick 'n' mix approach, with products from different ranges and brands, because you're more likely to get a broader range of key ingredients this way. But it's not a negative to use an entire range – just check that you're not paying for seven products with the exact same active ingredients as each other, for example all vitamin C or all antioxidant skincare. Skincare should be like a balanced dinner plate: a little bit of everything is needed. Just remember: chopping and changing too soon into a regime, not taking photos to compare and having little patience is usually more the 'issue' at hand!

Can I cleanse four times a day?

This is a super common question – as in, can I cleanse in the A.M., before the gym, after the gym and in the P.M.? The answer is that it depends on the cleanser. With a mild, nourishing, balancing cleanser that doesn't strip, a.k.a. dehydrate, the skin, it's fine, advisable in fact, and salicylic acid can be used (in low amounts) to remove the oil and sweat thereafter. With a foamy wash, I'd advise against it as a daily occurrence as it may remove the oils from your skin and leave it tight and irritated. In a nutshell, once the cleanser is kind and gentle and active cleansing is only used as part of a P.M. regime, that is ideal.

Is double-cleansing a myth to sell more cleanser?

Always my favourite question! Unfortunately, no, not a myth. Double-cleansing does have true tangible benefits, in my opinion, and it has been a recommended feature of a facialist's professional regime for many a year. Your first cleanse at night cleans the skin and removes makeup, SPF (no excuses), oil and debris. Your second cleanse at night will remove any residue and treat or nourish the skin by targeting a specific concern, such as dehydration, congestion, clarity, and so on. Double-cleansing ensures absorption of active ingredients for better results. Even if you don't wear makeup, physical pollution particles and SPF need to be cleaned thoroughly from the skin. Bonus: products you apply thereafter will be able to penetrate more efficiently once you've double-cleansed. It's like when you have eaten a delicious Sunday roast, and the gravy and all that tasty goodness is coated onto the plate. A quick swipe of the plate isn't going to remove everything, you need washing-up liquid to break it down thoroughly. A pre-cleanse will remove the majority, but you need to follow it up with something that will further lift oil and debris from the skin and ensure it is clean.

Is it all about actives?

Like 'clean skincare', 'active ingredients' isn't a regulated term. When I say it, I use it to mean ingredients that effect change in the skin somehow – for example, vitamin C and its collagen-boosting, brightening properties, or lactic acid and its exfoliating skills – once delivered at the right percentage, with the correct base formula and correct delivery systems.

If our whole routine was 'active', even by my standards there would be jobs not getting done. We don't need active ingredients to remove our makeup, prime our skin or counterbalance the effects of acids and retinols. Nonetheless, there are 'inactive' or 'passive' (essentially never irritating to anyone) ingredients that actually do a lot, such as prebiotics or ceramides. A well-balanced skin routine will include a balance of active and passive ingredients.

Can I use retinol plus other forms of vitamin A?

Yes! The main forms of vitamin A you'll find in skincare are retinol, retinyl palmitate and retinyl acetate. Ideally, I encourage all to use retinyl palmitate first, rather than going directly into retinol, predominantly just to avoid the acclimatisation process associated with retinol. To me, retinyl palmitate is the holy grail. I opt for a progressive approach to its introduction and maintenance.

There's no one timeline that works for everyone when it comes to introducing more vitamin A, which is why I'd recommend speaking with a skin expert on this.

How long will it take to see results from my skincare routine?

You're not going to like this answer, but it's honest. The average skin cycle – the process in which new skin cells are made and dead skin cells are shed from the skin – is 28 days, or one full month. But note that this varies depending on skin ageing, health and other factors, which means it could range between 25 and 34 days. Usually, hydration is visible instantly, textural differences show within 3 days, and true long-lasting results take 28 days plus. That is not to say that your skin will be exactly where you want it after 28 days, but more that there will be a measurable difference versus the progress picture you took on day one.

When it comes to changes made internally, some skincare supplements say 16 weeks or longer, because they rely on the maintained amount of a specific nutrient being in your system, and the data states similar. Always follow trial expectations. However, in my experience, essential fatty acids, such as omegas, have an impact within a week as they are assisting hydration. Similar to externally, it is easily impacted.

Where should I spend the most money in my routine?

Your serums usually do a lot of heavy-lifting, so this is where I'd allocate the guts of a budget. Serums tend to be pricier than cleansers or basic moisturisers, for example, because they manage to combine great potent ingredients, effective delivery methods and copious benefits in one – this combination truly tackles skin concerns. But if you are budgeting, choose affordable on everything else and invest in a good, multi-tasking serum as they have a smaller molecule size for better absorption of actives. SPF is skin health so in terms of priorities of what to spend on, it's just as important as serums. To summarise, a cleanser, a potent antioxidant-based serum and an SPF will set the correct foundation for a regime and also for results within the skin.

Can you decant your skincare?

It's fine to decant mild cleansers, moisturisers and the likes for travel. Be warier of active ingredients, though, specifically vitamins C and A, as they tend to be sensitive to light and oxygen. The same goes for acids. And don't ever decant your SPF – SPF ingredients are highly sensitive to light (in order to perform their role of protecting the skin from excess light) and you don't want to think you're being sun-savvy when you're accidentally not.

Please know that a large part of a product's testing phase includes making sure the packaging chosen is fit for purpose – colour, material, durability in heat, cold, altitude … be aware! Beyond the prettiness of the packaging, there is nerdiness that works to secure the efficacy of the active ingredients.

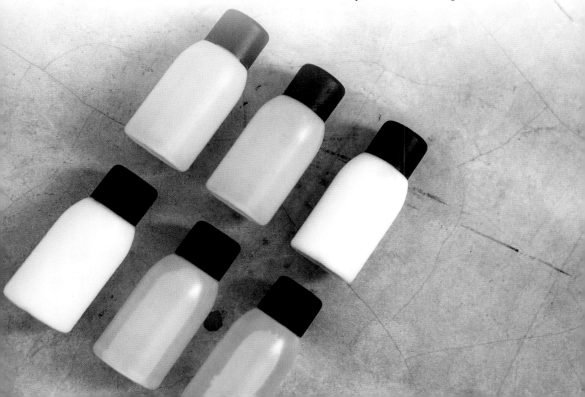

Should I gift skincare or is it best not to?

Don't gift active skincare unless you know the person and what they use very well! If gifting skincare to someone, opt for the type of product that will have a benefit for everyone's skin without there being potential for the product irritating their skin, for example hydrating mask, spritz, mild cleansers, SPF, hyaluronic acid and antioxidants. Steer clear of exfoliating acids, vitamin derivatives or anything 'ageing' – it's not very polite, unless they have specifically requested it. Anti-ageing under the Christmas tree – not for me! A cute spritz or sheet mask is always a diva winner! Skincare or skin consultation vouchers are great gifts too.

Are homemade skincare recipes a good idea or a no-no?

I'm not an advocate of homemade skincare in general. There are some shocking ideas out there of what's 'good' for your skin and I've seen my fair share of gritty homemade face masks and uber-drying homemade moisturisers. It ain't pretty, and I wouldn't recommend it. It's important to understand which ingredients work, in which combinations, and which ones should never be put near your skin – lemon juice, specifically, is a no-go.

Are scrubs ever okay? What about on my body?

Disliking scrubs can be a bone of contention in the industry, as scrubs can split opinion. I don't endorse them for the body or the face because, in my experience, chemical exfoliants for the body are much more effective.

Imagine dead skin cells as old roof tiles that you want to remove.

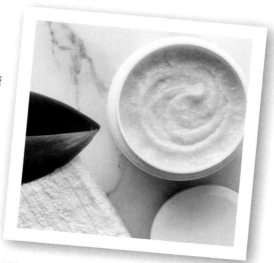

Chemical exfoliation (using acids which remove the dead skin chemically rather than physically) is like dribbling a mild solvent through roof tile cracks to help dislodge the already loosened tiles, rather than chipping them off from above. In this respect, chemical exfoliation, when used correctly, can be much gentler than scrubs. Interestingly and worth noting, the skin is acidic so all we are doing is using acid to our advantage – like with like.

Two scrubs I will say are fine … at a push … are lip scrubs (so long as the grain is superfine) and foot scrubs for the heels and calluses. Your feet are denser-skinned around the heels and are prone to calluses, due to friction, therefore making them somewhat more tolerant. I still opt for chemical exfoliants on my feet – have you tried the Footner foot peels or Baby Foot? Not the most attractive, but so satisfying to see the skin across your entire foot peel off after two weeks! But be aware that this is excessive and not to be performed unless the skin is visibly thickened.

Skincare tools

Why do professionals rub product in their hands? Should I do this?

No slick science-y reasoning here. It's just to spread the product easier or to warm it up before they put it on your skin. Professionals heat the product to ensure there's enough slip as the entire hand envelops the contours of your face or decollete, and they don't want to drag the skin. The less hand rubbing you do, the better, when you're dealing with active skincare, as it means that your hands aren't absorbing all that goodness. Your hands probably don't need 2 per cent salicylic acid!

When applying oils, body moisturisers and products that need slip and are covering a larger area, a professional tip is to place the product into the palm of the hand, put your hands together and twist them clockwise, then anti-clockwise, to gently distribute the product without rubbing it all over your hands. Always try to use the entire palm, fingers and indeed whole hand to contour and mould the area of the face or body to which you are applying the product. Typically, heat and pressure also have benefits in product penetration, and heat also provides circulatory benefit and, depending on pressure applied, lymphatic drainage, too.

Do electrical skincare tools work?

Home tools for EMS (electrical muscle stimulation), sonophoresis (sound waves) and iontophoresis (electrical current) are great for toning, increasing product penetration and boosting circulation and glow. FaceGym and NuFACE are known for their EMS Slendertone-for-your-face machines and Environ's Focus Care Skin Tech+ Electro-Sonic DF Mobile Skincare Device is a belter for assisting larger molecules (like peptides) penetrate further than hands alone allow. Similarly, the TT Skincare by Teresa Tarmey massage tool is ideal to aid in product penetration. As a facialist I will always be pro modalities (tools). The hands cannot be underrated or undervalued, but for product penetration and vibrations, etc. the technology in electrical skincare products is advancing rapidly and must be researched and respected. Results are a-comin'!

Do facial rollers actually do anything? Should I use jade or rose quartz?

The act of facial rolling for alleviating puffiness goes back to ancient times. Today's rollers are small, hand-held devices with jade or rose quartz stones and look a bit like mini paint rollers. Stone rollers make it easier to assist with lymphatic drainage to alleviate puffiness, but the same results can be achieved with manual massage. Rollers are just that bit handier, and act as a prompt and a reminder. Their cooling action helps to temporarily constrict blood vessels to get rid of that just-woke-up under-eye puff a lot faster, too, and using the roller typically means you will be more rhythmic in your approach. Remember, it is key to roll in the correct manner, i.e. towards the lymph node. On the neck, for example, this means rolling lightly downwards (no pressure is needed as the lymph is in a superficial situation, needing no pressure to activate it) as opposed to the traditional cream application technique, which teaches us to apply upwards. The lymph around the eye should be drained towards the front of the ear (towards the parotid gland), and then from the back of the ear to the lower central neck (from the posterior auricular to the submandibular gland).

From our perspective, there's much of a muchness between jade and rose quartz when it comes to depuffing and lymphatic drainage.

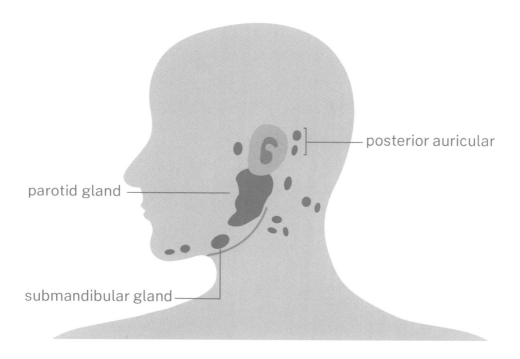

How do I keep my shower tools hygienic?

This one is a real toughie. It's certainly not easy. Hanging them outside the shower rather than leaving them lying at the bottom of the shower is ideal.

With anything you use in the shower, including cleansing bars or shower bars, the most hygienic thing to do is to dry them off after use and store them in a dry room rather than in the steamy bathroom. Steam + moisture = bacteria's 5-star hotel room. If you won't go to this level of effort, hang them within your shower, pat them dry and replace them as frequently as you can.

The most hygienic and sustainable shower tool is … drum roll, please … your hands. Who would have thought it? I use old Cleanse Off Mitts as shower tools to give them a new purpose, too. It's very handy to keep them clean as you can just put them in the washing machine at 30°C once a week. Change them regularly, do not wait for the annual Christmas giftset to receive the one loofah per annum! No comments needed – enough said!

The Fourth Nerdie Principle

Inform Yourself

Inform yourself. Yes, that's it, a short one. You need to be fully skinformed to make the best choices for your skin, so ask your questions, research your particular needs, take notes, keep a skin diary to chart your own progress and triggers, and invest that bit of time and energy in yourself because you'll be so glad you did. No question is stupid, no condition is shameful or embarrassing, no worry is silly – don't scold yourself, just go out and find the answers, be it through a book like this, or a skin consultation or your GP, who can refer you on to the relevant professional, if needed. Once you know, you can apply in practice – and that's a skin-saving measure!

Chapter 5

Your Skin Misconceptions, Unravelled

We've worked through the common questions people ask about skincare and that leads us nicely to the common misconceptions that are doing the rounds and have become accepted by many as inarguable truths. From the many hours spent talking to clients within the Nerd Network, I've realised just how much mis-skinformation is out there, and it can really get in the way of identifying the best-suited ingredients, products and routines for your skin. The wealth of facts and figures – and downright lies – ricocheting around the place make it easy to pick up a baseless piece of advice and treat it like it came written on stone tablets and must be obeyed – on pain of death. Harbouring misleading ideas can be detrimental to your skin health, so it's important to call out the common misconceptions and drag them, kicking and screaming, into the light to have a good look at them. So here's your guide to what's True and what's a Big Fat Lie (BFL).

Partly
TRUE

Not always. Undereye dark patches are often genetic. It is true that tiredness will make them worse – let's face it, it rarely helps anything – but the main culprits are genetics, thickness of skin under the eye, sun exposure and pigment type.

If you have deep-set eyes and thin skin around the orbital bone which surrounds the eye, you are going to have dark circles as a result, and there really isn't much you can do to change that. As your skin thins with age, the tissues begin to break down, which will make those dark circles more pronounced.

Some things will make a small difference, but nothing will get rid of these dark circles entirely, I'm afraid. You are trying to thicken the skin so that the blood pooling below your eyes won't be as noticeable, so the fat-form of vitamin A (retinyl palmitate) in a serum will begin to help over time. SPF is essential, and a mineral concealer will help to cover them.

I'd also recommend caffeine as a good measure because it can boost blood flow underneath the skin to brighten up the area and help prevent blood from pooling, which exacerbates that darkness. And no, I don't mean start filling the cafetiere and glugging. Take your caffeine in a serum or an eye cream – The Inkey List have a caffeine product, and the Kennedy & Co. Eye Gel contains caffeine plus a heap of antioxidants.

The root problem could also be pigment-related. The pigment in this under-eye area can be increased by UV rays, adding to the dark shading. For this you can use brightening ingredients like azelaic acid, vitamin C, brightening peptides, and liquorice root extract. Vitamin A is particularly effective here too as it works to assist in plumping the tissue and therefore, due to collagen and elastin synthesis, decrease the appearance by increasing the depth of the skin in that area. My personal suggestion for this type of dark circle, if it is something that really bothers you, is PRP or platelet rich plasma therapy. I've had it done and can vouch for it. In PRP, your own blood is taken, spun around to separate the plasma and then the plasma is injected back into you. This works to put your skin in healing mode and to provide it with growth factors, creating fresh skin quickly and reducing the appearance of the pigmentation. Many are dubious, but I've lived it.

A separate eye cream is essential

Partly **TRUE**

Eye creams split opinion: some experts rate them highly and see them as an anti-ageing essential whereas others think they are a marketing ploy. My opinion? I think that, for the most part, your undereye area can get what it needs from your serums and other products, so long as they are safe for use around the eye area. Lash that vitamin A, peptides, hyaluronic acid, ceramide-y goodness onto the browbone, under the eyes and around the outer corners. The pro-eye cream side often state that the eye area is more delicate and needs different amounts of actives. I beg to differ, provided the molecular sizing of your usual moisturiser/serum is correct so that it can penetrate into the skin, and the PH is tolerable, meaning it doesn't cause sensitivity. (A skincare expert can best advise you on this.) And not all eye creams are the same – some lower the amount of active ingredients to appease more sensitive eye skin, and others increase them because the eye area tends to age slightly faster than the surrounding skin.

If using an eye cream, make sure that the formula is different to what's in the other products you're applying to your face – otherwise, it's a duplicate purchase that isn't needed.

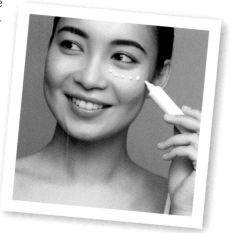

However, if you have tried the serum route and want more results, adding an eye product that is high in vitamins A and C and peptides may give you the boost you're looking for. I like the Environ Youth-EssentiA Vita-Peptide Eye Gel and the IMAGE Vital C Hydrating Eye

Recovery Gel. And don't forget caffeine – see the previous answer for more on that. Finally, less is more: use your ring finger to apply the cream in outward motions.

Eczema and psoriasis are skin conditions that can be 'cured'

FALSE

A total and utter BFL, unfortunately. Eczema and psoriasis cannot be permanently cured. They are lifelong skin conditions that require ongoing treatment and maintenance. There are peaks and troughs, depending on circumstances.

Eczema is also known as dermatitis and is familiar to sufferers as itchy, inflamed, swollen and crusty patches on the skin. The cell turnover is occurring too quickly in that patch of skin, leaving the skin more open to the elements, so it is a wound that is struggling to heal. You can't wash or scrub eczema away and its appearance is not your fault. There are plenty of topical creams to provide temporary relief, though I would strongly recommend probiotic skincare as it can have a phenomenal easing effect on the condition, as well as ingredients that can help with strengthening the skin, such as polyhydroxy acid. Gallinée have a great probiotic range and Skingredients PreProbiotic Cleanse is very gentle as well. It's also essential to include hyaluronic acid, antioxidants, vitamins A (non-retinol form), C and E and SPF in your daily skincare routine, to give your skin a complete helping hand in maintaining good health and wound-busting capabilities. But you also need to dig deeper into the root of the problem because it's often found inside your body – eczema triggers can include stress, diet and hormone levels.

Psoriasis is also a lifelong condition classified as a genetic, autoimmune disease. It's a very individual condition in that flare-ups will be different for each person, triggered by different things, although I regularly hear stress and alcohol listed as common triggers. With psoriasis, the skin is overproducing skin cells and in the process races to slough off 'old' cells to make way, but those cells are not ready to fall away. They then hang about on the skin's

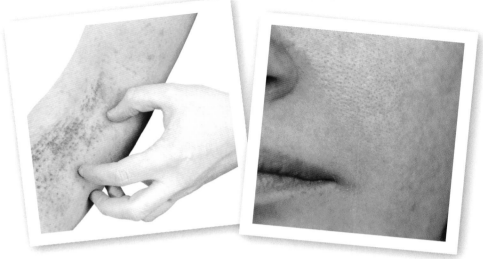

surface, clubbing together to form often large patches of scaly skin, which can be dry to the point of cracking and bleeding. Like eczema, this process creates a wound of the affected skin. In terms of treatment, all of the usual sensible advice applies – omegas, antioxidants, vitamins A and C and probiotic skincare. But psoriasis, like eczema, definitely requires medical assessment, so you need to pay a visit to your GP to assess your particular condition and explore the best treatment options.

Open pores are caused by popping spots

This one is True *and* False – just to keep you on your toes. There's a bit of a chain reaction involved here. First, what's important to understand is that pores aren't doors – they don't open and close – and they ain't a muscle either, as we said earlier. They are simply an opening, and how open is largely the luck of the draw. Some people have larger pores thanks to genetics, and those with oilier skin are more likely to have larger pores. However, open or large pores can be caused by trauma to the skin, such as popping spots poorly or popping spots that shouldn't have been popped in the first place. So it is true that spot-popping is one potential cause.

Another cause of large, open pores is cystic acne, which manifests as spots that never come to a head but are swollen, angry red and sore. They're no fun at all and can cause havoc with your pores. Cystic acne is produced by a consistent build-up of sebum, which leads to the pores becoming blocked and, potentially, the pore walls eventually collapsing, resulting in damage to elastin and collagen, meaning the pore doesn't have the same 'bounce back' elastin-wise and so it remains stretched. This can happen even when you've been sitting on your hands and not touching the spots at all.

Open pores can also be caused by skin laxity or loose skin, a natural part of ageing. Without you doing anything at all, the pores can become larger as the skin ages (from the age of 25 on) due to the degradation of the skin's structural proteins, collagen and elastin. The lowered levels of elastin again can lead to that loss of 'bounce back'.

So open pores are usually a chain reaction caused by genetics, maybe some manual zit-zapping, the overproduction of oily sebum forcing the pores wider and the effect of time marching ever onwards.

What can you do about it? Obviously keep your spot-popping fingers away from your skin. Plus I recommend you don't use blackhead strips or toners that promise to close pores, I'm afraid. Instead, be consistent with your skincare, use vitamin A to help strengthen the skin, and SPF and antioxidants will help prevent accelerated ageing. If you have the budget and time for treatments, opt for microneedling, which stimulates collagen and elastin production in the skin, helping pores to appear smaller. I am only an advocate of that, however, if vitamin A and the core ingredients are used in advance to assist skin health, results and, in turn, downtime.

Fake tan blocks pores and causes breakouts

Partly **TRUE**

Brace yourself: it's half a BFL. There are two types of fake tan: one is makeup, so it's simply applied onto the skin; the other contains DHA (dihydroxyacetone), which causes the Maillard reaction (the collision of amino acids, reducing sugars and heat, producing a caramelising or browning effect) and stains the skin. You eat the Maillard reaction when you fork a cooked steak. So when you apply DHA-containing fake tan, it's basically like basting yourself on a BBQ!

While the fake tan itself isn't a pore-blocker, there is some truth in the statement because of the human factor. Because people are keen to protect the tan, this can cause them to cleanse the skin less thoroughly or exfoliate less often. So if you're constantly complaining about fake tan giving you spots, just remember that a bad workman always blames his tools!

The Origins of Fake Tan

You might never have considered where fake tan came from, but it's a story of curiosity rewarded. Eva Wittgenstein was a researcher in America in the 1950s, working with children with metabolic disorders. The medication she was giving to her patients contained DHA and she noticed that when drops fell on the bed linen, nothing happened (which seems hard to believe, given how my bed sheets look!), but they stained the skin. Her researcher's brain wondered about this, so she rubbed some of the medication on her own skin to see what would happen. Lo and behold, her skin stained a light brown. Eva then had the genius idea of using DHA to give her legs 'tights' because nylons were in short supply.

Eight glasses of water a day is necessary for healthy skin

Partly TRUE

It is true that water hydrates the skin and is important for getting rid of waste and toxins as well, but you can drink water until the cows come home and it will make very little noticeable difference to the skin if you aren't also eating your essential fatty acids (EFAs).

As we covered in the How to Eat for Skin Health section, drinking water without eating EFAs is like putting up a shelf without brackets – it won't stay put. Without EFAs repairing cell membranes, the skin won't hold the water long enough to benefit from its hydrating effects. So that means eating a well-balanced diet of oily fish, nuts, fresh vegetables, grains and seeds, alongside drinking one to two litres of water per day. Additionally, the advice that drinking gallons of water detoxes you and will get rid of acne … BFL. Drinking plenty of water is beneficial for the skin, but acne is a complex skin disorder that requires multi-pronged treatment.

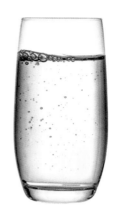

Blocked pores are caused by oily skin

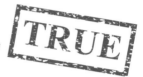

True! Yes, this one is bang on the money. Sebum, the skin's oil, is made up of lipids such as triglycerides and squalene and forms part of the skin's protective acid mantle, which makes the skin waterproof and keeps it lubricated. Therefore, sebum is very important, but our glands can over-secrete it and that's when the pores can get blocked with excess sebum. If this is an issue for you, there are various treatments you can try. Most people with blocked pores will find that salicylic acid works well. As it can be easier to control the effects, I recommend salicylic predominantly in wash-off formulations, such as IMAGE Clear Cell Clarifying Cleanser, the Murad Time Release Blemish Cleanser and the Environ's Clarity+ Sebu-Wash Gel Cleanser, as well as (of course) my own Skingredients Sally Cleanse. Some acids are oil-soluble and some are water-soluble, and oil-soluble salicylic acid is the main acid recommended for oilier skins. Other skin types may respond better to glycolic acid, lactic acid and polyhydroxy acid which are water-soluble.

If your skin really dislikes acids, it will tell you by feeling more touch-sensitive after application, perhaps not after the very first use but after a few uses. In that case, look into enzymatic exfoliants as an alternative approach (see box on the next page for more info).

The best treatment to improve the health of each pore is vitamin A, which can notably reduce the appearance of open pores. Another option is a clinical peel or treatment as this will truly penetrate beyond where homecare products often can and, speaking on behalf of skin facialists, we adore extractions on blocked pores. Oooh yes. There is a way to perform extractions properly, and we know it!

Enzymatic Exfoliation

If this is a new one on you, a brief explainer: enzymatic exfoliation is when we use enzymes – such as papain, which comes from papaya, or bromelain, which comes from pineapple – to exfoliate the skin. Enzymes are deemed non-irritating, a very gentle form of exfoliation as they can only 'gobble up' the deadest of dead skin cells. Enzyme products are typically smooth to the touch (no granules or grains), have no tingling effect and are effective when used regularly. Two I would recommend are the IMAGE Vital C Hydrating Enzyme Masque and the Declare Soft Cleansing Enzyme Peel.

Facial wipes are the perfect way to remove makeup effectively

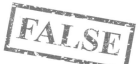

Wrong, wrong, wrong, all kinds of wrong. BFL alert! My immense dislike of wipes has been well documented, but it's always worth repeating because their efficiency is a tenacious idea. We have road-tested this at Nerd HQ by taking a hit for the team and using wipes for 14 days straight, just to double-check our facts. So, I can tell you that it is a fact that wipes strip and dehydrate and that they don't clean thoroughly, leaving debris to clog up your now mightily irritated skin.

I created the Cleanse Off Mitt (COM) as a reusable, convenient and affordable alternative that is very kind to your skin while cleansing it thoroughly. We know this because, as readers of *The Skin Nerd* might recall, we also conducted the Jesus Christ Test at HQ, so called because when you see the makeup left on the towel, you might exclaim 'Jesus Christ!'. This involves putting a white towel to the face after cleansing, to see how much debris is left behind. We check the inner lip corners, inner nose, back of the ears (your mother was right!) and the hairline, as these are the tell-tale places where you'll find the remains of makeup. After cleansing with wipes, you basically get the Shroud of Turin. After cleansing with the COM, you get a nice white towel. I'm not saying that's you completed on the cleansing front. It's just one part of your routine, but it's certainly superior to wipes in that it's alcohol-free and highly effective.

Cellulite is caused by weight gain and eating the wrong foods

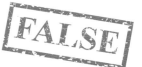

That's a BFL right there. The truth is that we all, no matter our body shape or type, have fat in our bodies. It's natural and it's here to stay. Cellulite occurs when fatty pockets protrude into the skin's tissues, causing the dimpled, puckered effect you often see on the magazine stands when some unfortunate celeb has been photographed in harsh sunlight in her bikini. I say 'her' quite deliberately, because it is especially common in women. Don't you just love being female? The joys. Women's connective tissue, which lies just above the subcutaneous fat, has larger openings, making it easier for the fatty protrusions to poke through. And naturally, it occurs more on the fatty areas of the body – take a bow, bums, tums and thighs.

And you can't cream cellulite away. Any cream that makes that claim is telling a BFL – a cellulite cream may assist in improving the skin's appearance but the effect will only be temporary.

There are things you can do to reduce its appearance, though.

Body brushing won't get rid of cellulite, but it will improve circulation and lymphatic drainage and help keep skin hydrated. Well-hydrated skin shows fewer flaws, so the cellulite will be less noticeable. The best time for body brushing is just before you step into the shower. It provides light exfoliation and gets the lymphatic system awake and working.

There are also mechanical massages available that can target circulation and lymphatic drainage. Endermologie Lipomassage and radiofrequency are both helpful in the battle against cellulite. (A cellulite cream can be used in conjunction with body brushing and massage.)

Alongside these, exercise, diet and water intake are also very useful allies. A 20-minute walk a day provides a great boost to the lymphatic system and circulation. But you don't get away that lightly. You should also work out two or three times per week to tone your body, which will reduce the appearance of cellulite. In terms of diet, your cellulite will thank you for eating food rich in antioxidants, vitamins and minerals. So think whole foods, natural foods, unprocessed foods – you know the drill.

Ageing is inevitable so it's a pointless waste of time and money to try to counter it

FALSE

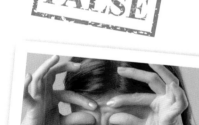

Yes, it's true that ageing is inevitable – and in my opinion, that's beautiful, because living long enough to grow older is a gift that should be wildly embraced. The thing is, we all harbour a desire to age gracefully when it comes to our skin and that can be harder to achieve. The problem is accelerated ageing, where our skin ages earlier and faster than it should, due to factors including stressors, smoking, poor diet and lack of exercise.

How do you know if you are experiencing

accelerated ageing? Well, there are no hard and fast rules because we are all, of course, skindividuals, but here's a rough timeline with regard to ageing and the skin:

- **25 years of age** – your skin stops producing as much collagen, which leads to fine lines and wrinkles, open pores and capillary breakdown (capillaries have less collagen in their walls and can collapse more easily, which can lead to broken capillaries and spider veins). At this stage, lines and wrinkles will not necessarily be deep-set or visible on your skin.
- **30 years of age** – the skin is slowing down, so it's making fewer skin cells and not exfoliating itself as quickly. Collagen and elastin continue to decrease. It is likely you can now see fine lines around areas of expression, like the forehead, lips and eyes.
- **40 years of age** – these lines may be visible even when the face is passive. There's now a rapid decrease in collagen production, which means skin looks less plump, less dense and the skin around the nasolabial (nostril to side of mouth) area may droop. You can likely see hollows and creases forming and the nasolabial crease is becoming more pronounced. Skin laxity is also becoming more pronounced, possibly with sagging around the jawline.
- **60 years of age** – for people who have menstruated, your oestrogen has probably now left the building, leaving your skin high and dry. Hydration and moisture are now key concerns. Fine lines may be increasing and deepening. Skin laxity continues to deteriorate, meaning the skin sags more, as its elasticity is becoming depleted.

These, whether you like it or not, are the norms of ageing skin. If your skin roughly corresponds to these markers, you're strolling towards a nice vintage. If your skin is hitting these markers earlier than the years given above, you could be experiencing accelerated ageing. Look at your peers, then assess how you are ageing by comparison. Are your lines and creases deeper? Is your jawline less defined? Do your frown lines remain furrowed for longer without animation?

Does your skin look a little bit rougher, redder and discoloured? If you are nodding 'Yes' to some of these questions, that points to accelerated ageing. But fear not, it's nothing to weep about. We will all age at different rates. This is not my way of encouraging you to analyse endlessly, simply an initial barometer.

The good news is that you can definitely fight accelerated ageing and it's not pointless to try. Your skin will still age according to genetics, but approximately 20 per cent of our skin's ageing is caused by extrinsic factors, which means you can take control of the degradation pace by making good lifestyle choices. If you want healthy-as-possible skin as you grow older, don't smoke, drink in moderation, exercise regularly and feed your skin a diet rich in antioxidants, vitamins and minerals. You also need to take control of your skin regime and tailor a Personal Action Plan for now and into the future.

If you wish to target accelerated ageing, you should do everything in both columns (unless directed otherwise)

How to target chronological ageing	How to target accelerated ageing
SPF EVERY DAY! Start this as early as possible and keep that habit going for life. (SPF is covered in more detail later in this chapter.)	Take particular care to avoid excessive sun exposure and absolutely wear SPF EVERYDAY.
Include vitamin A serum in your daily routine – it helps to prevent and reduce the appearance of fine lines and wrinkles. Start using this from your twenties and don't stop. (After daily SPF use, this is probably the single best piece of anti-ageing advice.)	Consider progressing along the vitamin A step-up trail.

How to target chronological ageing	How to target accelerated ageing
Include antioxidants in your diet and your daily skincare regime to help to protect from causes of inflammation. They are considered to be specifically anti-ageing because they help slow down the degradation of collagen and elastin. These include vitamins A, C, E, B3, green tea extract, liquorice root extract and resveratrol.	Apply topical antioxidants and UV protection daily to prevent damage from light and free radicals. Drink less caffeine and alcohol, eat less sugar. If you smoke, work to kick your habit. You can do it!
Take vitamin C supplements and vitamin A supplements – ideally, start doing this around age 25.	As well as vitamins A and C, consider taking an antioxidant supplement for added internal environmental protection.
Hyaluronic acid is essential for plumping the skin and keeping it supple – it's a massive water magnet that pulls water up from the skin's lower layers – but our ability to make it decreases as we get older so it's important to apply it topically. This acid can also pull water from the environment around you – but in areas of low humidity, where this isn't possible, the skin can get dehydrated if the acid is not locked in with a ceramide-rich product, such as a serum or moisturiser. Nerdie note: hyaluronic acid itself is not the game-changer, but hydration is key internally and externally, so it is an important factor.	The best forms of hyaluronic acid serum are those that combine different types of hyaluronic acid for longer-lasting hydration, deeper hydration and surface hydration. Bigger molecules can't penetrate as deeply so provide surface hydration, whereas smaller molecules can travel deeper into the epidermis for deeper hydration. Combos of cross-linked plus low-molecular plus high-molecular hyaluronic acid are best, like IMAGE Skincare Ageless Total Pure Hyaluronic Filler. Alternatively, your hyaluronic acid serum should provide other benefits, like a peptide and antioxidants, such as in Skingredients Skin Veg. Note that 1 per cent or more of hyaluronic acid in a formula is the known benchmark for results.

How to target chronological ageing	How to target accelerated ageing
From your thirties on, you need to get serious about exfoliation as skin is desquamating (shedding off naturally to make way for new skin) less. Always be careful not to over-exfoliate and don't use any product that's too gritty for this reason. Choose your exfoliating acid wisely. If you're working to tackle pigmentation, opt for lactic acid or PHA twice a week, depending on the formula. Or you could use glycolic acid every third night, again depending on the percentage of glycolic acid used, its PH and its base formula. Nerdie, much?!	Exfoliation is key – you can use a stronger exfoliation product but best to consult with a skincare specialist before doing so.
Peptides are the wunderkinds of anti-ageing and can have many functions, but the most commonly praised and used are peptides that promote the creation of collagen. They occur naturally in the skin and are the skin's protein, strengthening and protecting. You can add them to your routine by using peptide-rich serums and/or moisturisers.	Including peptides is of particular importance to those who may be experiencing accelerated ageing.
Body brushing and facial massage are ideal ways to improve circulation and stimulate the winding-down lymphatic system from top to toe including the face. We have many a facial massage demo on our social media.	Body brushing and facial massage is recommended for you too!

How to target chronological ageing	How to target accelerated ageing
As we age, our skin's natural hydration depletes and menopause can often mean drier skin (due to a drop in the hormones that regulate sebum production).	Hydration is very important for you too!
	Opt for Skingredients Skin Good Fats, Neostrata Skin Active Dermal Replenishment, Codex Beauty Bia Facial Oil or the Nunaïa Nourishing Radiance Serum. The last two truly massage the muscle while nourishing.
Post-55, it's necessary to introduce creamier, more hydrating cleansers, preferably with lipids which work hard to keep moisture in the skin.	The Nunaïa serum and the Codex Facial Oil are my choice for truly massaging the muscle while nourishing with such an anti-inflammatory oil.

You might want to consider a specialised treatment that is specifically designed for anti-ageing. The four I would recommend are:

* LED – this light treatment can stimulate the connective tissue (fibroblast cells) and produce collagen. It helps improve the tone and texture of the skin.
* Ultherapy – boosts collagen and reduces appearance of sagging skin.
* Microneedling – gets collagen growing and working.
* Electrical muscle stimulation – targets muscles underneath the skin to help stave off sagging and crepe-y skin.

Keratosis pilaris (KP) can be exfoliated away

FALSE

BFL, I'm sorry to have to report. These are the tiny red bumps commonly found on the back of the arms (but can be found anywhere on the body), often called 'chicken skin'. They are caused by a build-up of keratin in the pores, the result of an overproduction of keratin. The bad news is this tendency to overproduce keratin is genetic so it can't be changed or 'fixed'. But don't despair – there are measures you can take to tackle the little blighters.

Vitamin A is a good place to start because it is believed to help address the problems with the keratinisation process. Take it orally along with omegas to get a head start on preventing the build-up from occurring. You should also include acids in your skincare routine on any parts of the body affected – glycolic, salicylic and lactic – because they can be highly effective at softening the keratin and helping the skin to slough off dead cells that are clogging pores. Salicylic acid is a Rock Star Ingredient when it comes to KP – because it is oil-soluble it can penetrate the follicle and encourage cell desquamation at a faster yet gentle rate. Finally, hydration will also help to get the skin's processes humming along nicely. For this, you need hyaluronic acid and ceramides – look for them in the ingredients list of moisturisers and face creams. Topical vitamins A, C and E are additionally fantastic for KP.

Fear not if you have keratosis pilaris on the buttocks or upper thighs – it's common. Mechanical exfoliation is simply scratching the surface – literally. The keratosis pilaris originates deeper in the skin, so using a combination of an acid cleanser short-term to help dissolve plugs and a vitamin A-based reparative cream will do more than just hydrate the rough surface.

Stretch marks are only caused by pregnancy

FALSE

Nope! Stretch marks are caused by gaining or losing weight and by growing taller. It's not just a baby bump that stretches us out of shape. Stretch marks can also be caused by muscle growth, so they are relatively common among dedicated gym-goers. Finally, there's that word we all hate to hear: genetic. Yes, they can simply be the luck of the genes draw. There is no product that can erase stretch marks, but if trying to treat them, the key is to catch them early, while they are still red and fresh (i.e. while blood is still circulating). You could massage a vitamin A body cream or oil such as Environ ACE Body Oil into the skin daily, but this is not suitable during pregnancy – if pregnant, normal body oil or stretch mark oil is recommended. Topical treatments don't work alone, in my experience, so ignore any creams telling you they can banish stretch marks, although they may reduce the appearance aesthetically. The stretched skin requires specialised treatment.

As for older stretch marks, which are white or silvery grey in appearance and may dip inwards like a groove, at this point the scar has been 'sealed'. You may see some effects from stretch mark oils but you could also look into treatments that target collagen and blood flow such as microneedling or laser therapy.

SPF should be worn daily

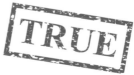

Yes, yes, yes! True! It is one skincare rule that you should treat as if it was written on a stone tablet and fell from the skies. SPF EVERY DAY! I can't say it often enough or loudly enough. It's crucial. It should be a key step in your skincare routine and you must never skip it – even if the heavens are chucking it down outside, you still have to wear SPF. Think of SPF like your knickers – a must-wear!

Excessive sun exposure causes sun damage and is extremely ageing to the skin, but sun is not the enemy – being sun-savvy is key. And it's not just the sun – it's all light. We have to protect our skin from light because it harbours UVA. This stealthy assassin penetrates the skin more deeply than UVB (because of its longer wavelength) which means it damages the skin's key structural elements, such as collagen and elastin (which can contribute to deeper lines and wrinkles and a loss of elasticity in the skin) and plays havoc with pigmentation. Our skin requires protection from UVB (present in heated sunlight) in the summer months, and UVA all year round.

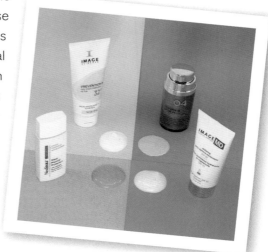

Choosing the Correct Sunscreen

Recently, the use of sunscreen has come under scrutiny following a report in the *Journal of the American Medical Association* (JAMA) regarding the absorption of certain ingredients into the bloodstream. The report wasn't saying this was a reason for concern, it was saying that it does occur and that more research is required to determine if this absorption poses any health risks. Inevitably, the headlines screamed panic, making people worry about what was happening every time they rubbed sunscreen onto their skin.

First, I'd like to reiterate that wearing sunscreen is an essential part of a healthy skin routine. Yes, you need to be happy with the ingredients in your chosen product and happy that your skin likes it, but once you are, you really do need to apply it every day. And in terms of the level of daily protection, you should choose an SPF of between 30 and 50. Some experts suggest lower SPF levels reapplied more frequently but my concern is that often people don't reapply as often as is required (according to the advice of the Irish Cancer Society). I endorse applying higher SPF protection evenly to protect as best you can.

So how do you choose the best sunscreen? There are two types: chemical and mineral/physical. It's the chemical sunscreens that received all the bad press, so I'll start with those. Chemical SPF works by initiating a chemical reaction that converts the UV rays into heat and then releases that heat. Oxybenzone, octinoxate, octisalate and avobenzone are all forms of chemical SPF filters. These sunscreens tend to be light and thin, so you need less of them for good coverage, which is a plus point. On the minus side, they take about 20 minutes to kick in and start protecting the skin, they can irritate the skin or result in an allergic reaction, they can clog the pores of those with oily skin and they require regular reapplication to keep them working at optimum levels. The concern provoked by the JAMA report centred on how much of these chemicals are absorbed through the skin into the bloodstream. (The effects of this absorption are not yet known.) However, oxybenzone scored highest for absorption and researchers are wary of its effects, given the results of initial studies – additionally, oxybenzone has been found to cause damage to coral reefs. So the current recommendation is to steer clear of this particular ingredient until further research can supply a decisive answer to the question of whether or not it has an adverse effect on the body.

The mineral sunscreens take a different tack: they stay on top of your skin, like an angry sit-in protest against the sun, and they deflect the rays away from the skin. This is why they are also called physical blockers. The main ingredients of these are titanium dioxide and zinc oxide, which are active mineral UV filters. Studies have shown that these do not seep into the bloodstream, they start working as soon as applied and are better for sensitive skin and heat-activated skin. Thanks to all these plus points, mineral sunscreens tend to perform better in tests to ascertain safe and efficient screening from the sun's rays.

My Skingredients SPF is mineral, because upon speaking with tens of thousands of Nerd Networkers, I learned the vast majority would prefer to opt for this type as it is less likely to cause sensitivity or irritation, and it starts protecting immediately – I know that hoomans are an impatient lot at times!

You might be thinking of the thick white difficult-to-rub-in sunscreen your mother slapped on you, but fear not. The range of daily SPFs available today are designed to be worn under makeup and are lightweight and moisturising to boot. When applying, always follow the recommended Skin Nerd approach of nipples up: start just above the nipples and press it gently into the skin of the chest, neck and then face – essentially, anywhere you are exposed. It's easy to buy cheap sunscreen in the supermarket, but this won't necessarily give you the full protection you're looking for in terms of your skin's health – antioxidants for pollution protection, HEV, and infrared. I've included tips on reading the labels along with my top recommendations in Chapter 6.

Liver/Age spots are caused by ageing

FALSE

Wrong. They are caused by sun damage. The lesson here is to apply your SPF from the nipples up and all across your hands. This will afford you protection from those creeping age spots, particularly if you spend a lot of your time driving, where your hands are facing up towards the sun daily.

Finally, while you may think I've lost the plot completely, be sure to apply SPF if you are inside all day but sitting in front of a computer screen. There is a lot of data for and against this theory, but many trials I have read conclude that there is an impact. Even though the roof is keeping the sun away from your skin, your screens (computer, phone, TV) are emitting high-energy visible (HEV) light – in other words, blue light.

My advice isn't that we should retire from our day jobs and never look at another electronic device again, but we should consider shielding ourselves from a form of light that many of us are exposed to for 40 hours or more a week at work. and more again at home. So find a daily sunscreen that suits your skin and wear it every single day. No excuses, Nerds!

The Fifth Nerdie Principle

Always and Ever SPF!

It's one of the cornerstones of skincare: wear SPF every day, without fail or exception. I never, ever start my day without SPF – at this stage, I can't even imagine life without that essential protection on my skin. If I went out without it, it'd be like one of those weird dreams where you're in a crowd and suddenly realise you forgot to put on your trousers. I would definitely end up in that kind of trouserless sweating panic if I realised my skin was going commando on the SPF front. SPF is the foundation of all your anti-ageing work, so make a habit of it.

Wrinkles are caused by the effects of ageing on the skin

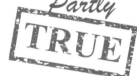

This is only true to an extent. Age can and does play a part, but wrinkles, or rhytides to give them their official name, have various causes:

* They can have a genetic basis.
* They can have a mechanical basis, i.e. repetitive expressions and motions, like smoking/vaping or sleeping on one side every night.
* They can have an environmental basis, thanks to sunlight and pollutants in the air.
* They can have a psychological basis, in that stress can make us pucker up and frown.
* They can have a dietary basis, as sugar molecules bind to elastin fibres and cause wrinkles that way.

Wrinkles are an inevitable part of ageing, and the worse news is that there are many things in your environment that can accelerate their development. Short of wrapping your face in clingfilm and never, ever smiling, you're going to have to accept your wrinkles – maybe it would help to see them as living memories, folded onto your skin, reminding you of all the times you laughed. Is that helping at all? Maybe not … Even though you can't keep them at bay forever, you can slow them down by following a few basic rules. Use SPF every day along with the best moisturiser for your particular skin needs and age, and eat a diet filled with skin-friendly vitamins. Especially … what vitamin? A! You know it! Eat it and apply topically.

There are so many causes of wrinkles that are simply not your fault, but one where I'm afraid the blame lands squarely on your shoulders is the drinkle. Stop wincing, you'll wrinkle! Drinkles, as we've already learned, are the offspring of dehydration (which increases the appearance of fine lines and wrinkles). Basically, if your skin is gasping for water, it's not likely to look its best. Thankfully skin is very forgiving, so once you rehydrate, it does wonders and diminishes the appearance of those drinkles. But when indulging in alcohol, go easy – for your skin's sake.

Smoking will accelerate the ageing process too, so if you do smoke, try to compensate for depleted vitamin C levels at least by eating plenty of vitamin C-rich foods and taking supplements, and maintain a healthy diet.

PROTOCOL:

How To Do Your Own Research Into Skincare Claims

The problem with doing your own research will always come down to source legitimacy. When searching online, any key phrase may bring you a wealth of knowledge from respectable and trustworthy educational sites (US university website addresses will end in .edu), but it also may lead you to the opinion of someone in their basement who has never learned a thing about chemicals in their life. Don't get me wrong, I don't have a degree in science myself, but my qualifications, years of experience and the advice of other experts assures me that I know which sources I can trust. If you want to educate yourself, you definitely can, so long as you follow these tips to help you sort the science from the unproven opinion.

If you're not that nerdie, follow the science nerds who make it easy

There has been a lot of backlash about beauty bloggers in the last few years. However, some beauty bloggers are cosmetic scientists who analyse research and let us know what the facts are, or who are opinion-led and encourage awareness that although a product may not be for them, it may be for you. These are the beauty bloggers I follow, and I recommend you do the same. Skincare is different from makeup – a red lippie can be judged immediately due to pigment and durability, for example, but that's less the case when it comes to skincare. Two of my favourites are Lab Muffin, a.k.a. Michelle, an Australian with a PhD in chemistry and a love for skincare, and KindofStephen, Stephen Alain Ko, a cosmetic formulator who curates the best beauty news, new studies and opinion-based beauty articles.

Doing your own research

If you like roaming around the internet, looking for things to grab your interest or to inform you, then do it mindfully – especially when it comes to looking for advice you're planning to follow.

Opt for websites:

- run by government bodies or reputable international organisations – in the UK, the NHS has lots of factual information on skin conditions, in Ireland, the HSE website is an excellent resource, and there's also the World Health Organization (WHO);
- run by skin foundations and charities;
- geared towards providing information to medical professionals, like the American Academy of Dermatology;
- universities or other educational facilities.

Finally, be wary of websites that seem like legitimate, government-based health resources but aren't – unfortunately, there are tonnes of them out there. Read their 'About' page to assess their background, agenda and methodology.

Some super-nerdie sources

- Irish Skin Foundation: general advice on skin conditions.
- Irish Cancer Society: a great source for knowledge on skin cancer and how to prevent it to the best of your ability.
- British Journal of Dermatology: publisher of high-quality dermatological research.
- American Academy of Dermatology: plenty of information about skin conditions, concerns and misconceptions.
- INCIdecoder.com: a search engine that allows you to find out more about ingredients.
- PubMed: a biomedical literature portal, useful for locating and accessing research papers and journals.
- Harvard Health Publishing: a concise source for information on anatomy, physiology, how the skin works and specific skin concerns.

If you're willing to get nerdier, you can interpret research papers

If you're not in college, nab your nearest student's JSTOR account (or any digital library, for that matter) and get searching. In Nerd HQ, we use PubMed a lot, which is a search engine full of biomedical literature from around the world. Simply type in your keyword or key phrase, keeping it as simple as possible, and get perusing.

There are a few things to keep in mind when you're looking for good results among research papers and literature reviews:

- the size of the trial being carried out – eight people versus 121 people makes a huge difference.
- the amount or form of any particular ingredient – trials usually test the efficacy of an ingredient in a specific amount suspended in other ingredients or formulated with other ingredients, and this may mean the data is not as relevant as you think.
- when it was carried out – more recent data is usually more relevant.

Don't just read the abstract of the paper. Read the whole thing, all the way down to the Conclusion, or use the Table of Contents to find the relevant section for your particular research concern.

There are some cons to doing your own research, though: it's more time-consuming and difficult, and you may misinterpret what's said at times. Also, there can be a tendency to treat research papers as gospel, but they're not always as unbiased as you'd think.

THE JOY OF EXPERT HELP

I am all for independent research, thinking and decision-making when it comes to skincare, but I also know that going it alone can be daunting and it can take longer to identify the best products and product mixes for your skin. This is why professional skin experts always emphasise the importance of an initial skin consultation, particularly if you are working to improve particular skin conditions such as eczema, acne, psoriasis, or skin issues such as wrinkles, oiliness or redness. When a skin expert examines and assesses your skin, they can quickly identify your primary and secondary issues and potential causes and can use that information to create a tailor-made plan for your skin, now and into the future. Beauty therapists are trained in anatomy and physiology, skin, skin types, skin care, skin diseases and disorders and treatments, and any Nerdie beauty therapist undergoes continuous training and education to remain up to date with new ingredients, modalities and findings on skin.

This is why we run the Nerd Network alongside the Skingredients range, because one optimises the other – and we are *all* about the optimising! You may have skin concerns but don't feel equal to the very large task of researching it all or may feel you're getting nowhere with your skin. If this is the case, then I'd strongly recommend a consultation with an accredited skin expert.

Chapter 6

The Skinvestigator

It's time for an in-depth skinvestigation into skincare products and their ingredients. It can be very difficult to keep up to date with developments as the major corporations strive to deliver the latest in skincare technology. In addition, if you pick up any product on your bathroom shelf – say, your current moisturiser – and look at the ingredients panel, you'll be confronted with a list of words that seem to come from another planet. Would you know if propylene glycol is a good thing for your skin? Aluminium starch? Disodium EDTA? Myristic acid? Cetearyl glucoside? Thought not. It's daunting, to say the least, and it reiterates the truly scientific element of skincare.

I have dedicated over ten years to deciphering this stuff and am quite the skin detective at this stage. On top of that, I spent two years creating and trial-and-erroring The Skin Nerd's own skincare range – Skingredients. Thanks to this very involved and fascinating process, I've gained a whole new insight into product ingredients and what works and what doesn't. (I've also gained some new grey hairs, but hey, what's a few grey hairs among Nerds?) I know the Rock Star Ingredients, the ones that are usually great for every skin type. And I want to share this knowledge with you –

knowledge that is essential to your own understanding and decision-making.

I'll take a simple and straightforward approach so that you don't fall asleep halfway through. My goal is to educate you so that you can read the INCI list (the ingredient list) on the back of the bottle, arm you with the knowledge to separate the marketing from the science and equip you so you know what is for and what is not for *your* skin. That way, you'll make the best decisions for your skin's lifelong health.

The product types

First off, let's look at how the product is described. You might encounter the words 'natural', 'clean' and 'active skincare' on the label and in the branding. What do these mean, exactly?

Natural skincare

This is an often hotly contested claim because there is no firm agreement over what exactly constitutes 'natural' and there are no standards in place to market a product as such. If you take 'natural' to mean natural to the skin/body, you would be wrong. Take witch hazel and tea tree oil as an example. Often touted as natural ingredients, they do exist naturally, but they aren't actually found in human skin or bodies. On the other hand, ceramides, squalene, hyaluronic acid, vitamin A, collagen, amino acids and peptides are all found naturally in the skin/body, but they haven't really been christened with names that reflect that. Is this what natural means – already existing in the skin/body? By that reckoning, witch hazel and tea tree oil get lobbed out of the natural gang, although that is not how the consumer often sees it.

The other huge concern I would have with this labelling is that people often take 'natural' to mean 'optimum', 'better than not-natural' – even if they're not entirely sure what 'natural' skincare is. Thanks to the power of marketing and suggestion, consumers can feel mighty virtuous if they bring home something with 'natural' written on the bottle. But often the ingredients that suffer under unwieldy names are stellar performers and necessary to healthy skin. Hyaluronic acid is a good example – yes, it has 'acid' in its name, but it's not exfoliating or drying. It is, in fact, a hardcore hydrator. It's a respected ingredient and earns its place in any well-rounded skincare routine.

So don't work from an unconscious bias when it comes to the word 'natural' – it doesn't necessarily mean better.

Clean skincare

Another hotly contested topic in skincare because there is no agreed, global definition of 'clean' and no requirement to prove a product is 'clean'. Clean skincare, as opposed to natural skincare, usually contains 'bioactive' elements, i.e. ingredients of botanical origin that can have a significant effect on the skin. Some retailers have created their own guidelines to help consumers, such as the Clean At Sephora initiative. Most brands will be declared 'clean' if they're free from certain nasties, usually including, but not limited to, parabens, SLS (sodium lauryl sulphate), petroleum by-products, synthetic fragrances, silicones and chemical preservatives. But this doesn't mean that all other products are 'dirty'. As we've already seen, there are natural ingredients that can irritate some skin types, so don't fall into the trap of reading 'clean' as 'superior'. Clean beauty products can be great and highly effective, and I admire any company that takes steps towards this concept, but it's not the case that 'clean' means it's the perfect product for you.

Active ingredients

I have already shared my vision for the bright new world of skincare – the Skin Active Movement – and active skincare certainly has a part to play in that. 'Active' means containing ingredients that can cause a change in skin condition. (Sometimes active skincare is known as cosmeceutical skincare, but this is not a regulated term, and all skincare technically falls under the umbrella of cosmetics.) The most common active ingredients are alpha-hydroxy acids (AHAs), salicylic acid, vitamin C, retinol, hyaluronic acid and peptides.

There was a time when active skincare was exclusive to salons and clinics, but now you can find active skincare on pharmacy and department store shelves, including products from brands such as Drunk Elephant, The Ordinary, The Inkey List, Kate Somerville and our own Skingredients. Their active status warrants education on the pack (and any claims should have scientific evidence to back them up) as well as a level of nerdie support thereafter. Active skincare can be a culture shock to the skin if it doesn't come with education on how it should be used correctly, so I always recommend starting small and building up.

It's worth noting too that many cosmetic skincare products don't contain high percentages of active ingredients but still have a place in any skincare routine because they tend to be more nourishing and texturally comforting.

The ingredient types

The many ingredients you'll see listed on skincare packaging can be subdivided into their distinct types: acids, antioxidants, hydrators and brighteners.

There are also solvents, preservatives, pH balancers and other ingredients that many class as 'filler ingredients', i.e. ones that don't directly benefit the skin but are vital for stability, viscosity and other factors. These 'filler ingredients' are integral to how a formulation will work.

Acids

These often get bad press because, let's be honest, there's something about 'acid' that sounds aggressive. This is terribly unfair on the acids because they work their compounds off to deliver good skin results. And they sound much scarier than they are. For example, if a label says vitamin C, you're straight in there, 'I'll have some of that, thank you very much', but if you read ascorbic acid, you might be hesitant. However, they are in fact one and the same thing. So the word 'acid' does not inherently indicate 'bad' or 'stripping' or 'drying' – acids are actually of huge benefit when used correctly in a stable formula that does not allow oxidation.

In skincare the most common acids are alpha-hydroxy acids (AHA), beta-hydroxy acid (BHA) and polyhydroxy acids (PHA), all forms of exfoliating acids that can be used in lieu of mechanical exfoliation. When you see these in the ingredients list, they'll often be simply given as glycolic acid, lactic acid (AHAs), salicylic acid (BHA), and gluconolactone and lactobionic acid (PHAs). I consider these – particularly salicylic acid, or Sally as she's known to me because we've been friends for so long – to be Rock Star Ingredients. You need them to help with skin that's dull and sluggish, ageing, acne-prone and/or sensitive.

AHAs are particularly good at bringing about skin-smoothing and speeding up skin cell turnover, and as a result can be very beneficial for pigmentation, lines and wrinkles. Lactic acid is hydrating, and has a larger molecular size than glycolic acid, so is more suitable for sensitive skin. Glycolic acid has a smaller molecular size than other AHAs, meaning that it can travel deeper into the skin for a more intense exfoliation. Salicylic is *the* chemical exfoliant for oily and acne-prone skin because it not only encourages the skin to slough off pore-clogging dead cells, but as an oil-soluble acid it can 'get into' the pore and dissolve sebum and debris. It's effective on blackheads, whiteheads, lumps, bumps and under the skin spots, from the tip of your forehead all the way to your bum (yes, I do care about bum spots, too!). PHAs are the second generation of AHAs. They are basically just like AHAs, but more suitable for reactive skin and inflammatory skin conditions.

One of my go-to glycolic acid products is the Neostrata Foaming Glycolic Wash (with 18 per cent glycolic acid and 2 per cent PHA) but it is strong, so not for exfoliating acid beginners. For some salicylic acid recommendations, turn to page 123. PHA is harder to find as a stand-alone exfoliator (you can find it in Skingredients Sally Cleanse and PreProbiotic Cleanse) but The Inkey List have a PHA Toner that comes very highly rated as an exfoliant for sensitive skin.

The other heroic acid that must be mentioned here is hyaluronic acid. Unlike the others, it's a hydrator, able to hold up to a thousand times its weight in water. In spite of its intimidating name, it's gentle enough to be used on baby skin (in the right doses!), and it hydrates without oiliness or heaviness, so it's generally suitable for all skin types. To get that hyaluronic acid in, I would choose Skingredients Skin Veg, IMAGE Skincare Ageless Total Pure Hyaluronic Filler or The Inkey List Hyaluronic Acid Serum.

Takeaways

- Acids are friendly, often naturally occurring chemicals that benefit your skin when used correctly.
- Your skin is acidic, so fear not, applying an acidic skincare formulation has advantages once the short-term impact it may have on your skin (such as potential dryness or flaking) does not detract from the long-term results. (Note: don't apply them to broken skin or to your lips as the acid will irritate those areas.)

Antioxidants

These ingredients, which kick the ass of oxidants, are essential for skin protection and long-term health. Oxidation, caused by free radicals, occurs when too much oxygen reaches a specific area and causes damage. I always use the apple analogy here: you know when you see an apple's flesh turn brown after someone has taken a chunk out of it and then left it sitting on the kitchen counter for someone else to clean up? Well, that's oxidation. Exposure has accelerated the amount of oxygen getting into that patch of flesh and it has caused free radical damage.

When you translate this process to human skin, the effect of oxidation is to create an army of free radicals that damage the DNA of the 'mother cell', or keratinocyte, which in turn damages the cell membrane and the DNA of the nucleus, making the skin cell less healthy than it was. Over time, this compromises the overall skin health, including depletion of collagen and elastin and damage to the skin's barrier function, reducing healing capacity and leading to sluggish skin cells, making the skin more vulnerable to sensitisation and light damage from various sources – sunlight, blue light, pollution, etc. The annoying bit is that sitting naked on the kitchen countertop isn't what causes oxidation of the skin – that would be easy to remedy. Instead, we are besieged by a number of different sources of oxidation damage, such as smoking, stress, a not-so-healthy diet, alcohol, unrestful sleep and air pollution. If we don't want the apple on the counter to go brown, we must put lemon juice on it, and antioxidants perform a similar role in skincare.

Respecting the Mother Cell

Keratinocyte is a bit of a mouthful. It's also basically a type of skin cell that makes up around 90 per cent of the epidermis. These cells divide to create new cells – hence the 'mother' bit because they generate new cell life. However, if the DNA of these cells becomes damaged by pollution, smoking, alcohol, etc. – our usual rogues' gallery – then they lose life force and can't do their job as well. It's the vicious mother cell circle: unhealthy skin creates more unhealthy skin.

Nothing can stop oxidative stressors, such as light and pollution, from affecting our skin, but we can work to limit the damage. And the good news is that you can launch a two-pronged attack on the free radicals by taking antioxidants internally and applying them externally. You can eat your antioxidants in a healthy and balanced diet by hoovering up lots of leafy green vegetables, fruits and green tea. You can apply your antioxidants directly to the skin with targeted active skincare – some potent antioxidants include vitamins C, A and E, niacinamide (vitamin B3) and green tea extract.

Green tea delivers an almighty dose of polyphenols, which are basically free-radical head-hunters. Polyphenols are also anti-inflammatory, so they help to bring down the redness and irritation associated with various skin conditions, such as psoriasis, eczema and problematic skin. So drink the green tea and apply the green tea extract for maximum antioxidant warfare.

Takeaways

- Antioxidants fight a major battle on your skin's behalf.
- You can boost their effectiveness by taking them internally and externally.

Ceramides

Plump, dewy, youthful skin – if you're living that dream, ceramides can take a lot of the credit. Ceramides are one of the lipids (fats) that help to make up our skin's natural moisturising factor (NMF), a layer that keeps the skin plumped up and acts as a protective barrier. It's a warrior on our skin's behalf, but – and it's a really big but, I'm afraid – from your thirties onwards your ceramides are beginning to pack up and leave town. Our natural process of ceramide creation starts to tail off, and that's what leads to thin skin, vulnerable skin and ageing skin. Research has shown that people who have dry skin and those who have conditions like eczema and rosacea have lower-than-normal levels of ceramides. Our skin needs their defence and protection efforts, which is why moisturisers are fortified with ceramides – especially those designed for older skin. They are an essential and recommended part of your daily routine, so choosing a ceramide-heavy product is a really good idea.

There are different ceramides you'll find in products, including ceramide NP, ceramide EOP, ceramide NS, or phytosphingosine and sphingosine. We included ceramide NP in Skingredients Skin Good Fats, and CeraVe as a brand takes its name from ceramides – their Hydrating Cleanser contains three of the skin's essential ceramides along with hyaluronic acid. You can also eat your way to higher levels of ceramides by chowing down on soy beans, eggs, dairy, wheatgerm and brown rice.

Takeaways

Our skin benefits hugely from the work of ceramides, but they decrease rapidly as we age. This makes them an essential addition to your skincare routine to combat the signs of ageing, and potentially help with itchiness and irritation in the skin.

Peptides

Peptides are linked amino acids, and by linking together in certain ways they create proteins. They are like the skin's post office, firing off messages and instructions between the cells. For example, they can send signals to the dermis to up collagen production, which is a message you want to get through loud and clear because it helps to reduce wrinkles and fine lines. Peptides share some of the skin-enhancing qualities of ceramides, such as fighting skin laxity, reducing the effects of ageing and working to preserve the skin's youthful texture. There are too many types of peptides to list, and many are patented blends, but most ingredient names will have the word 'peptide' in there, such as palmitoyl tripeptide-5, copper tripeptide-1, or dipeptide diaminobutyroyl benzylamide diacetate, or hydrolyzed soybean fibre (a notable exception to the 'peptide in the name' phenomenon).

Takeaway

Peptides are bossy boots ingredients which send signals to the dermis to carry out functions or trigger specific processes. Most types of peptide we see in skincare work to brighten the skin or up collagen production, but peptides serve many purposes in skincare.

Brightening ingredients

These ingredients brighten the skin's appearance by working on areas of discolouration and evening out the skin tone, so are an excellent solution if you have pigmentation issues. An excellent soothing and brightening ingredient is liquorice root extract. On the label it might be called glycyrrhiza uralensis, glycyrrhiza inflata or glycyrrhiza glabra, but they're all still plain old liquorice root extract. It is a pigment synthesis inhibitor, which means it stops the creation of pigmentation by collaring tyrosinase, the pigment-creating enzyme.

Vitamin C is also a potent brightener that works to inhibit tyrosinase, as is niacinamide, another name for the water-soluble vitamin B3. These brightening ingredients often have a big role to play in active skincare to address the effects of specific skin conditions such as hyperpigmentation and post-inflammatory hyperpigmentation, but they also have a place in a daily healthy skin ritual and I recommend you incorporate them into yours, especially if you are looking to improve uneven skin tone or 'age spots' (see pages 97 and 126). Ageing is as much about discolouration as it is lines and wrinkles.

Takeaway

Brightening ingredients help to boost skin radiance and reduce the effects of ageing.

Hydrators

There are three key types of hydrator:

* Humectants: ingredients that bind water to them, for example hyaluronic acid, glycerin and honey.
* Emollients: ingredients that soften the skin's upper layers and create a film across it, for example shea butter, fatty acids, grape seed oil and jojoba oil.
* Occlusives: ingredients that create a film across the skin to lock in moisture, for example silicones like dimethicone and squalane.

There is overlap in these categories, in that an ingredient can be two at the same time, but all three types may have a place in your skincare routine. Humectants and emollients are important for all, but those with dry skin will need more emollient ingredients and those with very dry or sensitive skin will need more occlusive ingredients.

Takeaway

All skin types need hydration – even oily skin – and our lifestyles make it incredibly easy for our skin to not be as hydrated as it should be, so it's essential to have multiple types of hydrators in our skincare routines.

Boo, hiss! The 'bad rep' ingredients

There are some ingredients that have been elevated from the obscurity of the ingredient listings and become famous – for all the wrong reasons. Even though most people couldn't explain what they are or what exactly their misgivings are about them, they'll say, 'Oh I don't use them, they're bad.' But when pressed to explain their thinking, they can't tell me precisely why, and the role of marketing (or anti-marketing) may be at play here. Or an ingredient might be toxic or have negative effects in large doses but very helpful effects in small ones. It's an unsupported 'certainty' that has filtered down from some unspecified source and acquired the status of truth. I caution all of my clients to be wary of this – if you believe something, ask yourself why you believe it and if you can't give yourself a solid answer, look it up and find out if you're right or wrong. Here, we'll investigate a few of the most common skincare 'villains', and I'd like to give you an objective view that might challenge your thinking. (For more on this topic, see page 263.)

Parabens

Essentially, no one had heard of these until a study conducted in 2004 (see page 263) put them in the headlines. The contention was that parabens could mimic oestrogen and could potentially lead to breast cancer. It became relatively common to see '0% alcohol, 0% parabens' on skincare and beauty aisle products as manufacturers rushed to reassure rattled consumers.

So, what are parabens? Chemically, they are a series of a naturally occurring acid known as 4-hydroxybenzoic acid, but when used in skincare they are usually synthetic and work as a reliable preservative.

The study that suggested a link between parabens and cancer was subsequently questioned because of inconsistencies in the methods used. A second study examined the link and found it to be inconclusive. So the current stance of the scientists is that there is no proven link between parabens and cancer, therefore they are safe to use. In spite of this, the bad feeling around parabens has lingered and I have found that even when I explain their backstory, my clients still prefer not to use skincare products containing parabens. That's why my Skingredients range uses other forms of preservatives. But from my own reading and research, I can see no reason to be scared of parabens.

Another side-effect of the tide turning against parabens is the rise of substitute preservatives that haven't been researched very much. If you check your ingredients list and satisfy yourself that there are no parabens present, but the product has a shelf-life of 12 months, what's doing the work of keeping out microbes and preventing mould from forming? There has to be a preservative present in the mix. The most common replacement preservatives at the moment are derivatives of phenols, which are very attractive because they are effective, affordable, natural and good at their job, but they have been studied less than parabens have. The potential problem with natural preservatives like phenols is that generally they have to be used in higher concentrations than their synthetic cousins in order to be as effective. These higher levels can irritate some skin, even though the phenol used is 'natural'. So you're getting the 'paraben-free' product that gives you peace of mind, but the alternative isn't necessarily better.

Sulphates

Sulphates have had a bad rep for quite some time, and none more so than sodium lauryl sulphate (SLS). You'll find them in skincare products because they are effective cleansing agents – they're the chaps that produce the satisfying foaminess of many products. They are classed as a surfactant, which means they attract both oil and water. Their molecular makeup means that one portion cuts through water and the other cuts through oil, and that double whammy removes dirt and oil from your skin or hair. That's why you'll find SLS and other sulphate types listed in skincare products, soaps, shampoos and cleansers.

So far, so good, so why the bad rep? There was a study in the 1990s that linked sulphates to cancer. Multiple studies since then have disproved this alleged link, but the ghost of that hypothesis has hung around sulphates ever since and it makes people nervous when they see them listed as an ingredient. My only issue with sulphates is that they sometimes do their job too well and strip away so much oil that skin can become irritated or reddened and hair can become dry and brittle. But I don't believe they are massively less drying than sulphate-free products. I would recommend avoiding sulphates if you have shown an individual sensitivity to them, but otherwise, there's no need to be wary.

Scents

Can you recall the scent of your mother or grandmother's moisturiser, or her perfume, or talc? Most of us can – it's a strong smell association and can trigger vivid memories. That scent came from the parfum added to the product for that exact reason – to create a scent that the wearer feels is 'theirs' and that enhances their use of the product. You might be massaging in a moisturiser, but if it has a gorgeous scent, a whole other sense is involved and the experience is more pleasurable. Scent is the only reason parfum is added to skincare – it performs no other function. It masks an unpleasant smell and may hide an oxidised 'off' scent as a product matures. This is why many people feel it's an unnecessary addition and prefer to go without.

The key question is, of course: what is parfum? It will be on the ingredients list as natural parfum, parfum or fragrance – but other scents found in skincare may crop us as citron, limonene or an essential oil, for example. Parfum is often a blended mixture and you won't find its constituent parts listed, which means you can't know as the consumer what that fragrance is made up of.

If you find that a fragrance of any kind, whether an unlisted blend or essential oils, irritates your skin, seek out fragrance-free skincare products. My own Skingredients range is completely scent-free – as my motto goes, 'smells don't change cells'. So I look to perfume for scent, not my skincare products. (Perfumers may cry, but I spray perfume onto my clothes rather than onto my skin as the high alcohol level can irritate it.)

PEGs

They prefer to be addressed as polyethylene glycol, but they're just PEGs to me. Primarily a surfactant, they have a whole host of uses in skincare because they can work well on their own and also play nicely with other ingredients. PEGs have impeccable manners. They are often mixed with hydrating emollients (soothing, softening substances) to create gentle cleansers, and also form a great team with fatty acids and cleansing agents.

As a result, PEGs form the basis for a wide array of products, including moisturisers, cleansers and sunscreens. You'll often see them on the ingredients list as PEG-100 stearate. This labelling indicates that they are serving as an effective emollient ingredient – the kind of thing you want in your moisturiser. An emollient creates a non-oily, breathable coating across the skin that forms a defensive barrier and locks in moisture. PEGs are also emulsifiers and can be used in cleansers to help oils on the skin to mix with water so they can be easily removed. The extra bonus is that PEGs are non-irritating and non-toxic.

The flip side of this is that there is a lot of unease around PEGs based on the idea that they could be harmful. There was once a basis to this argument, when the manufacturing process was less sophisticated and created unwanted ingredients alongside the wanted PEGs, but this has long since been ironed out. The other angle on the bad press was that they were tested in high concentrations on animals. Again, this was true at a certain time in the past, but thankfully it no longer applies. Now, PEGs are a versatile, reliable ingredient that bring a lot of the oomph to your daily routine.

Ingredients and Pregnancy

You have to be mindful of what you're rubbing into your skin when you're pregnant because your skin might be extra-sensitive while you're growing a hooman. (P.S. Congrats!) Here is a list of products that should be okay to use and others to be wary of:

* Most skincare ingredients are fine for using during pregnancy, including hyaluronic acid, vitamin C, vitamin E, botanical extracts, peptides and SPF. As always, SPF is key as it can help to prevent excess pigmentation.

* Lactic acid is suitable during pregnancy for exfoliation, although because it is water soluble, rather than oil soluble like salicylic acid, it is not as effective at penetrating the pore to help with congestion. Niacinamide can also be beneficial for decongesting.
* As your skin can be more sensitive, you may want to be aware of products with fragrances.
* It's not recommended that you use salicylic acid as it is derivatively related to aspirin, which isn't recommended for use during pregnancy).
* Glycolic acid is suitable for use during pregnancy, but caution is required because it can lead to light sensitivity, which can contribute to melasma/chloasma (the 'mask' of pigmentation some experience during pregnancy)
* Retinol and vitamin A are not recommended for use during pregnancy, either internally via supplements or externally, although smaller amounts of vitamin A in products are sometimes approved for use during this time. If you're unsure, check the packaging or contact the brand.

Put Your Hands Together for the Rock Stars!

Rock Star Ingredients are the ones that really pack a punch and do mighty work on your skin's behalf. They are kick-ass, focused and persistent in fighting the effects of ageing and the many pollutants that try to drag your skin down. Here is a list of those skin heroes and we salute them! (Please note that this list is not in order of importance/effectiveness.)

- Vitamin A and derivatives, like retinyl palmitate
- Vitamin E
- Vitamin C, e.g. ascorbic acid
- Niacinamide
- Provitamin B5 – panthenol, improves skin softness and elasticity, ideal for skin's barrier
- Ceramides
- Hyaluronic acid
- Zinc oxide – mineral SPF filter with antioxidant qualities
- Tea extract, e.g. rooibos or green
- Lactic acid
- Polyhydroxy acids
- Glycolic acid
- Kojic acid
- Alpha-arbutin – usually extracted from bearberries, it's a potent botanical tyrosinase inhibitor
- Peptides
- Probiotics (e.g. lactobacillus) – for soothing
- Colostrum – in skincare, bovine colostrum is rich in growth factors that encourage skin healing and reduce inflammation.

The Sixth Nerdie Principle

This one's straightforward: education! It's my goal and my purpose in life and I want you to adopt it into your skincare routine. I'm not saying it's easy to find out and learn about the science of skincare, but it's a good investment in your skin to inform yourself as best you can so that you can make educated choices. Obviously, you already want to do this because you're reading this book, but I can't stress the importance of knowledge enough. There are lots of choices out there and lots of information to navigate, but education is like a ball of twine so that you can find your way at all times. That's what I'm doing – giving you a big old ball of twine to lead you towards Skinlightenment! And it doesn't have to stop here – this book will help to provide you with skin knowledge but you can continue the journey through online research, listening to podcasts, reading blogs, talking to a skin expert … there are so many ways to supplement your skin education.

PROTOCOL:

Skinvestigating the Ingredients Panel

So, you're in the shop or pharmacy or online and there they are, the gleaming rows upon rows of skincare choices. They all look good enough to eat, they all boast about their skin-changing properties, they all would look so stylish on your bathroom shelf. So what do you choose? Let's break it down a bit.

Now, I can't give you the list to end all lists and cover everything you'll ever see on a product label because that would require the death of more trees than I care to have on my conscience. But I *can* list for you the key ingredients, what they target, which skin types they work well on and my own tried and trusted products that contain them.

Ingredient	Ingredient type	Function
Glycolic acid	Exfoliating acid – AHA	Exfoliates dead skin cells with extreme effectiveness
Lactic acid	Exfoliating acid – AHA	Hydrates and speeds up cell turnover
Salicylic acid	Exfoliating acid – BHA	Chemical exfoliant for oily and acne-prone skin, dissolves dead skin cells and oils, is also anti-inflammatory
Polyhydroxy acids	Acid – PHA	More gentle than AHAs and BHAs, hydrating, increased cell turnover, antioxidant, can strengthen the skin
Green tea extract	Antioxidant	Attacks free radicals and therefore the effects of ageing, anti-inflammatory, brightening

Works well with this skin type	Names on label	Recommended products
Ageing skin, dull skin, sluggish skin. Must be used under guidance as it can cause huge change very quickly and be dehydrating (not recommended for sensitive skin)	Glycolic acid	IMAGE Ageless range, particularly the cleanser, serum and overnight mask, REN Glycolactic Radiance Renewal Mask, Neostrata Foaming Glycolic Cleanser and Peel Kits
Sensitive skin, ageing skin, dry skin, dull skin, sluggish skin. Much gentler than glycolic acid, so it's better for reactive skin	Lactic acid	Environ Derma-Lac for body and face, Skingredients A-HA Cleanse, Teresa Tarmey Skincare Lactic Acid Treatment
Oily, spot-prone skin, KP, bacne, bum spots. Not recommended for use during pregnancy, especially in high amounts	Salicylic acid	Skingredients Sally Cleanse, IMAGE Clear Cell range, Murad Time Release Blemish Cleanser
Good for those whose skin is sensitive to acids and therefore can't use glycolic or lactic acid	Gluconolactone, lactobionic acid	Neostrata Bionic Lotion, Skingredients PreProbiotic Cleanse, Skin Veg, A-HA Cleanse, The Inkey List PHA Toner
Ageing skin, dull skin and good for skin prone to redness or irritation	EGCG, epigallocatechin gallate, camellia sinensis leaf extract	IMAGE Ormedic Bio Peptide Serum, Skingredients Skin Protein and Skin Veg

Ingredient	Ingredient type	Function
Resveratrol	Antioxidant	Boosts body's supply of enzymes that battle free radicals, protection from pollution-related ageing
Hyaluronic acid	Hydrator	The boss of hydrators, stellar humectant
Vitamin A (retinyl palmitate)	Vitamin	Essential for healthy skin, repairs DNA damage, fantastic for fine lines, wrinkles, reducing oiliness, reducing congestion, improving skin hydration and helping to reduce the appearance of pigmentation
Vitamin C	Vitamin	Tackles pigmentation issues, antioxidant, strengthens capillary walls, reduces redness, helps skin to synthesise more collagen

Works well with this skin type	Names on label	Recommended products
It's a plant-derived antioxidant, so there should be no issues for any skin type	Resveratrol (*In Skin Protein and in some other serums, it may be a resveratrol-rich extract added so the ingredients listing may be, for example, polygonum cuspidatum root extract – which is Japanese knotweed.)	SkinCeuticals Resveratrol BE, Skingredients Skin Protein, Caudalie Resveratrol Lift Range
All skins but use is not advised in very dry environments as it may work to further dehydrate skin by pulling moisture outwards	Hyaluronic acid, sodium hyaluronate	Skingredients Skin Veg, IMAGE Ageless Total Pure Hyaluronic Filler, The Inkey List Hyaluronic Acid Serum
All skin – it's the first building block of healthy skin	Retinyl palmitate (other forms of vitamin A include retinol, retinoic acid, retinyl acetate)	Skingredients Skin Protein, Environ AVST range
Skin that needs excellent anti-ageing care and skin with pigmentation issues	Ascorbic acid, ascorbyl tetraisopalmitate, magnesium ascorbyl phosphate, retinyl ascorbate, tetrahexyldecyl ascorbate, ascorbyl glucoside (among others)	Skingredients Skin Protein, Skinceuticals CE Ferulic, IMAGE Vital C Range, Murad Essential-C Cleanser, Environ Radiance+ Intense C Boost Mela Even Cream, Neostrata Enlighten Range

Ingredient	Ingredient type	Function
Vitamin E	Vitamin	Softens, moisturises, antioxidant, protects from UVA damage, hydrator
Peptides	Cell messenger	Boosts collagen production, reduces effects of age
Ceramides	Skin-native lipid	Improve skin hydration, and are believed to assist the skin's barrier due to their role in its makeup
Kojic acid	Brightening	Targets pigmentation, acne marks and age spots
Liquorice root extract	Brightening	Stops the creation of pigmentation, antioxidant, soothes, brightens
Vitamin B3 (niacinamide)	Brightening	Works to reduce age spots and acne marks, brightens, reduces appearance of fine lines and wrinkles, helps with skin laxity

Works well with this skin type	Names on label	Recommended products
Dehydrated, dry or mature skin. Note that it can clog pores of those with oily skin, so use in small doses in this case	Tocopherol, tocopheryl acetate	Skinceuticals CE Ferulic, IMAGE Vital C Hydrating Antioxidant ACE Serum, Yon-Ka Vital Defense, Environ AVST 1-5, Skingredients Skin Protein
Ageing skin	Palmitoyl oligopeptide, acetyl hexapeptide *Some patented peptides will appear on INCI lists as, like with Skin Protein, soybean fibre, for example	Neostrata Skin Active Firming Collagen Booster, Environ Youth EssentiA Vita Peptide Eye Gel, IMAGE Ormedic Balancing Bio-Peptide Crème, Skingredients Skin Veg and Skin Protein
Dry skin, dehydrated skin, irritated skin, ageing skin	Ceramide NP, ceramide AP, ceramide EOP, ceramide NG, ceramide NS	Skingredients Skin Good Fats, CeraVe, Neostrata Dermal Replenishment
Dull skin, skin with pigmentation issues	Kojic acid	Neostrata Enlighten Pigment Lightening Gel
Dull skin, ageing skin, skin with pigmentation issues	Glycyrrhiza glabra root extract, glycyrrhiza uralensis root extract	IMAGE Iluma Intense Lightening Serum, Skingredients Skin Veg
Ageing skin, skin affected by inflammation, dull skin, skin with pigmentation issues, uneven skin tone	Niacinamide, nicotinamide	Murad Rapid Age Spot Correcting Serum, Skingredients Skin Shield SPF 50 +++ and Skin Good Fats

Ingredient	Ingredient type	Function
Parabens	Preservative	Help to keep a product fresh and free from bacterial growth
Sulphates	Surfactant	Incredibly effective at removing oil
Retinol	See vitamin A	Increases skin cell turnover, stimulates collagen production
Alcohol	Degreaser	Thins the product so it feels weightless on the skin

Works well with this skin type	Names on label	Recommended products
Those with easily irritated skin may need to avoid parabens	Methylparaben (E number E218), ethylparaben (E214), propylparaben (E216), butylparaben and heptylparaben (E209), isobutylparaben, isopropylparaben, benzylparaben and their sodium salts	Found in many cosmetic products
Those with sensitive skin, easily irritated skin or extremely dry skin may need to avoid sulphates if they irritate their skin	SLS – sodium lauryl sulphate, ammonium sulphate, SLES – sodium laureth sulphate, ALS – ammonium lauryl sulphate	Found in many cosmetic products
Ageing skin, pigmentation		IMAGE MD Retinol Booster, Neostrata Skin Active Retinol + NAG Complex, Murad Retinol Youth Renewal Serum
As it's a degreaser, often targeted at oily skin, but the truth is that volatile alcohols strip and dry the skin and weaken it and shouldn't be used by any skin types. These types of alcohol are essentially pro-ageing in high amounts and when they do not provide another purpose within the formula.	SD alcohol, denatured alcohol, isopropyl alcohol, methanol, benzyl alcohol	Found in many cosmetic products

Ingredient	Ingredient type	Function
Fatty alcohols	Hydrator (thickener)	Provide good texture and stabilise the formula; non-irritating, emollient
Glycerin	Hydrator	An effective humectant moisturiser, holds onto moisture and pulls moisture towards it
Sodium gluconate	Gluconic acid in salt form	Can neutralise metals in skincare (copper, for example), can be used as a pH balancer, softens the skin
Citronellol	Fragrance	A fragrance with citrus-like scent that is widely used in beauty products, including skincare; has antioxidant benefits but its skin-irritating properties negate these
Limonene	Fragrance	Very widely used in grooming products to produce a fresh, citrus-y scent, has antioxidant benefits but its skin-irritating properties negate these
Phenoxyethanol	Preservative	An excellent preservative to keep skincare products working at optimum level – the key to proper use and efficacy is the concentration level

Works well with this skin type	Names on label	Recommended products
Dry skin	Cetyl, stearyl, cetearyl alcohol, behenyl alcohol, isostearyl alcohol, myristyl alcohol	Found in many skincare products
Suitable for all skin types, especially dry skin	Glycerin	Many skincare products, including Skingredients PreProbiotic Cleanse, Skin Veg, Skin Protein, A-HA Cleanse, Skin Good Fats
All skins	Sodium gluconate	Found in many cosmetic products
Not recommended for those with easily irritated skin, or those who are allergic to fragrance	Citronellol	Found in many cosmetic products
Not recommended for those with easily irritated skin, or those who are allergic to fragrance	Limonene	Found in many cosmetic products
All skin types	Phenoxyethanol, 2-phenoxyethanol	Skingredients

Ingredient	Ingredient type	Function
Propylene glycol	Hydrator (preservative, solvent)	A humectant ingredient, which means it's a water magnet, and it also enhances how effective a formulation is, acts as a solvent and as a preservative
Disodium ethylenediamine-tetraacetic acid	Chelator	Preservative and enhances performance of the formulation

Works well with this skin type	Names on label	Recommended products
Not recommended for those with sensitive or easily irritated skin	Propylene glycol	Skingredients Sally Cleanse
In research on disodium EDTA, it doesn't irritate, sensitise or penetrate the skin	Disodium EDTA	Found in many cosmetic products

Chapter 7

The Story of Skingredients®

You'll be very aware by now that the science of skincare is complex, sometimes controversial and deeply fascinating. My nerdie sense tingles when I get skin-deep and truly tucked into this topic – there's so much to learn and so many possible permutations to create the right balance in any given product. I have been studying this science for more than a decade and in the last few years I have put my learnings into practice by developing my own range of skincare products: Skingredients. While I was working on my first book, I was also immersing myself in an intense learning experience as I worked with the team at Nerd HQ to design a clinical, yet attainable, reliable and effective range of targeted skincare products. It was a challenging and rewarding process. I am incredibly proud of what we've achieved and of the products we've designed from concept stage, especially now that I'm seeing and hearing about the results from the hoomans who use them. That is why I want to share the story of Skingredients with you here and give you the lowdown on what it is and what it does. I believe this will offer insight into the sector beyond ingredients and brand alone – and hopefully will offer you a small glimpse of the love behind the brand that thousands use daily.

I know this chapter lies in a section about what you should be doing when it comes to finding your own skin health solutions, and if I'm honest, I believe Skingredients could be a strong option for many a hooman. This skincare range is a physical manifestation of The Skin Nerd philosophy which is results-driven, with simplicity, education and expert help at its core – in short, efficient skincare that delivers.

The skincare vision

The idea of my own skincare range was hibernating inside me for a long time. The creative spark came from my 15,000-strong Nerd Network clients, whose opinions about their many different skinterests and insights I often seek out. It struck me that I was hearing the same words over and over again – active skincare, price, accessibility – so I knew the demand was there for my education-focused range. The skincare sector was confusing to many, saturated and overwhelming, so I wanted to simplify it. They wanted results, they wanted affordable options, and they wanted education through advice and support. I wanted to deliver all that, with noticeable skin improvements, within 28 days. I like to set the bar high!

I can tell you that creating a product line is a long chain of incredibly hard work in order to make each piece fit into the right place. The science behind it is unforgiving – achieving the balanced, active products I wanted to create was going to take a *lot* of trial and a bit of error. Once I had the vision for the Skingredients range, I met with 12 different pre-launch formulators from across the world – in Ireland, the UK, Germany, France and the US – to find the right partner. It was very hard to convey my vision because a capsule skincare collection that can benefit all skins and all hoomans with active ingredients is still relatively new in many markets. I needed a formulating partner who understood that the Skingredients range absolutely had to do what it promised to do – it had to be based on clinical data rather than jazzy marketing claims, packaging and smell.

The next step was to brief our top-choice formulators and ask them to create samples, which were trialled extensively at Nerd HQ. From this point, it took us two years pre-launch to be satisfied with the formulas; I always knew what ingredients I wanted, and the exact doses. I had to be sure that the formulations were made exactly right, with no money-led decisions affecting the quality of the ingredients. So after a lengthy testing process, I eventually chose two formulators to create different products within the range in the US and Ireland.

That was the single most significant part of the process completed, the part that was crucial, time-consuming and heart-breaking and the largest and hardest professional decision I've ever made in my life: what was inside the bottles, which was, as the name suggested, the optimum ingredients for skin health. I worked with an independent cosmetic chemist separate to the manufacturer's chemist to check all standards were met – even surpassed – and that we explored all options and how different ingredients worked in different formulations. We pushed to see all the ways that an ingredient could work within a product.

Then I had to think about what the packaging would look like, which is not as straightforward as you might imagine. The product bottle itself also needs to be tested rigorously: for compatibility with a solution, i.e. the temperature, how it sits, lies, flies, behaves in cold climates and warm weather, how it is pumped, how it is distributed when dispensed, how it dispenses when running low, whether the product will be air-pumped or not, how we could prevent oxidation – it was a relentless task. Before the products were submitted for toxicology testing and signed off by regulatory bodies, we carried out compatibility testing where the product is tested within the packaging, testing for different regions such as the EU, Australia and America, dermatological and ocular tests to ensure the products had been tested to dermatological standards and were safe for use around the eyes.

I wanted the packaging to be hygienic, clean, educational, colourful for a sense of identity, engaging and informative: I wanted the range to reflect our identity: fun, vibrant and unusual for the skincare sector. I opted for bright colours because I had realised that people often didn't remember product names, and it's easy to become confused by shelves of similar-looking products. Enter the idea of vibrant colour-coding, short names and numbering, giving three ways of remembering the products (depending on how your brain retains information) – so people who want the PreProbiotic Cleanse can remember it by name, or by its number (01) or by colour ('the purple one').

Naturally, you can't just pour cream into a bottle, slap on a pretty label and write some poetry on the side about how life-changing it is. Although that said, some brands do take a much easier route and buy a formulation already created, then place their logo and branding on it. This is called white labelling, but it was not the road for me because I wanted to make my own formula, from beginning to end – a harder task but one that has been worth it in the short- and long-term for all our clients and users of the product. I had noticed a need for ingredients in a certain blend, and I wanted to have full autonomy over every last ingredient, not just the key ingredients. My chosen route meant there was rigorous testing involved to ensure any products being brought to market are safe and reliable and that all claims placed on the bottle are not simply to entice buyers but are truly provable; there's also a responsibility piece when you are the brand founder and owner of the intellectual property both at a European accrediting body level and at Irish legislation level. It's a lengthy process and, I'll be honest, it was tough at times, but I knew it was there to protect people and guarantee high standards. The EU has very strict regulations around product claims and a 12-week stability test for every product as the norm. We also opted for premium, additional non-obligatory tests, such as ocular testing, comedogenic testing, dermatological testing. On top of all that, we're now doing further tests … stay tuned! It takes a lot of effort to tick every box, but we got there. And, more importantly, we will not stop there. As part of our philosophy to offer the optimum standard of product, we surpassed the norm of testing with more extensive testing due in 2021. What we're doing is not the norm and in large part makes no commercial sense, but we want *all* the facts – not just enough to satisfy our marketing. Nerdie facts and data are at the heart of all we do.

In June 2019, Skingredients was launched. It was one of the most remarkable moments of my life, making all the dreams, meetings, travel and personal sacrifice worthwhile. I was giddy and nervous with the anticipation of our clients seeing it, trying it and loving it. But I had confidence in the range because I had poured every sliver of knowledge, passion and first-

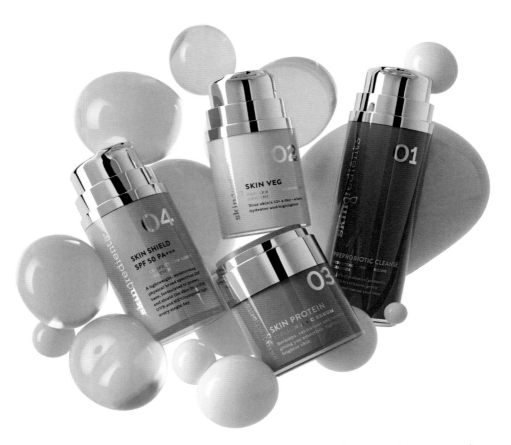

hand experience I possessed into the design, formulation and creation of the products. There is a new testing phase now because we decided to opt for university-led, independent clinical testing to prove the results delivered by the range. All in all, Skingredients was a two-year process from first brief to shelf. I know that may sound short, but the relatively quick production was down to the fact that it was a thoroughly well-thought-out concept before we embarked on the process. I wasn't following trends, every single thing about Skingredients – concept, protocol, ingredients, packaging decisions and manufacturing – was based on knowledge gained over years in the skindustry. I knew the ingredients levels, I know skin, I know my clients and I was confident that I could create what they deserved – skin health for all skins.

It has been a steep learning curve and an incredible journey ever since then. Month by month, week by week, day by day, we see more and more people converting to the Skingredients way of life and telling us about the results and benefits they have experienced. We had virtually no marketing budget, so it succeeded largely by word of mouth. We had hundreds on the waiting list, on pre-order, and that support shown by many of you reading this now has been mind-boggling, overwhelming and is not something I take for granted, believe me – it's deeply appreciated. This ground-up phenomenon made it even more satisfying to see Skingredients take off as it has. The capsule range of seven products might be small, but it really packs a punch. The range has been, and continues to be, thoroughly road-tested by the Skingredients users, who aren't shy about speaking their minds! Via department stores, clinic partners and hundreds of pharmacies countrywide, we receive countless queries and testimonials, especially as we work so hard to engage effectively with all of our customers and equip them with the know-how to – know how! If it didn't work, they would be shouting it from the rooftops. But, like me, they keep coming back for more because it does work and they can see the results. I'm so proud of what we've achieved with Skingredients, and unbelievably excited about the future and what else we can do. Watch this space! Or at least, go to www.skingredients.com so you can watch educational videos and use our live chat to ask your questions. It's a huge hub of information, and it's growing all the time.

✔ The Skin Nerd clients asked for active skincare – every Skingredients product uses proven ingredients, all painstakingly selected based on a targeted function. Tick!
✔ Our clients asked for affordable skincare – Skingredients hits a price point below that of many cosmeceutical products and spends less on marketing and endorsements to guarantee this affordable price level. Tick!
✔ Our clients asked for accessible products – I chose to distribute directly to salons and clinics, and use a second-party distributor specifically to give us access across a wide spectrum of retail outlets. As a result

Skingredients features in hundreds of pharmacies and department stores across Ireland (and will soon be in the UK too) that have been carefully selected – those that would invest time in training with our Head of Education, attend webinars and become Skingredients Nerds. The range is also one click away online through The Skin Nerd channels: theskinnerd.com and skingredients.com. Tick!

Those pharmacies, salons, department stores and clinics have engaged with Skingredients to an incredible degree. We hold monthly webinars to update them, and perform onsite and offsite training regularly to ensure they have all the knowledge available on the range. These partners have been phenomenal – to thank them all I would need ten more chapters! But this journey has taught me that loyalty and the support of independent and chain business owners is essential. It does not go unnoticed. We know that they help spread the message of skin health. These two-way conversations – with retail partners, Skingredients users and members of the Nerd Network – are key to us. To be honest, we were fortunate that so many outlets sought to stock Skingredients, and we were able to choose 250 partners we are honoured to work alongside. When you see Skingredients for sale, it means we trust that retail partner and they trust us.

The Skingredients® philosophy

I have worked for, alongside and with many different brands in many capacities, predominantly as an international trainer of products and treatments. This has allowed me to fall in love with lots of excellent products: there are so many brands I will never stop endorsing. So as much as we're very proud of Skingredients, I will always encourage hoomans to keep using what they are using if it is the right product for them, and this has earned us loyalty. We are not biased and happily recommend other brands.

The main driving force of Skingredients is education. It's not just about knowing how to use the range and what's in each product, it's about knowing

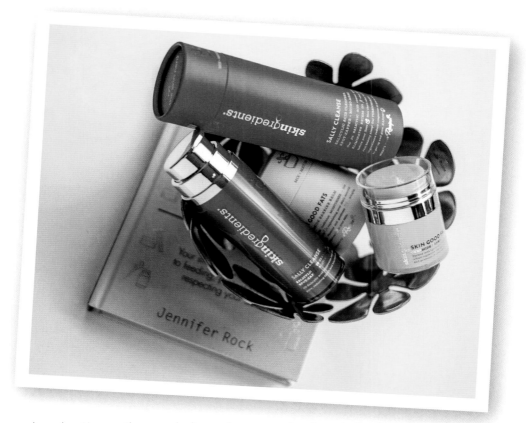

how *best* to use them and why you're even using them in the first place. That's The Skin Nerd in a nutshell – or a skin cell. And Skingredients is a range of active skincare products (with some products containing high amounts of active ingredients) so it's most important that clients are empowered with the knowledge they need to use them responsibly.

The education goal is there in every detail. There are infographics on the bottle giving you a step-by-step guide to how to use the product. There is a QR code (that matrix barcode you see on packaging) on each and every product with links to more information, including how-to-use videos for each one. There is a full ingredients list, with glossary (an explanation of each), on the bottom of each pack. No ingredient is omitted from the list or disguised in any way – just clear, comprehensive information. At Skingredients.com, our live chat and social media is manned by our knowledgeable team so that you can ask us questions any time you need to. There is a Skingredients Head of Education who travels to every stockist, giving expert guidance and advice so that they can give you expert care. This level of support – online webinars, articles, videos and manuals – is unusual, especially for a small start-up, but it's part of who we are.

The reason behind all this support and care is that I want our customers to really understand their skin in a holistic sense and, from that, understand the ingredients they need and therefore why the product is of benefit to them.

At the beginning of the book, I talked about the importance of a Personal Action Plan – but it's important to know too that taking action when it comes to your skin means respecting it and treating it with kindness.

The Skingredients®

Skingredients are comprised of vitamins, exfoliating acids, amino acids, prebiotics, probiotics, botanical extracts, fruit and veg extracts, good fats, minerals, anti-inflammatory teas and peptides that help to protect, nourish and maintain the skin, reduce and prevent the signs of extrinsic ageing and assist in targeting your skin concerns. It's the crème de la crème of what we find in nature and the powerhouse of lab-made ingredients that work for the skin. A lot of the ingredients featured are probably ones you've heard of before but you also probably have not found them in the custom-made combos we've created. It's this synergy of elements that gets results.

The name says it all, really. Skingredients is absolutely all about the ingredients – what's carefully put in. How they work together and complement each other is the key to the products' success. Skingredients focuses on what will normalise, brighten, hydrate, protect and correct the skin, assisting in oil control, hydration, barrier defence, tackling the depth of lines and wrinkles, redness, open pores and more. You'll find generous dollops of the Rock Star Ingredients, like salicylic acid, peptides, prebiotics, hyaluronic acid, vitamin A and vitamin C crammed in there. What you won't find is scent: every product is entirely fragrance-free. I was warned that not using 'smell memory' could impact the bottom line but because scents can cause irritation and sensitisation (and smells don't change cells!), I was adamant that skin protection and results had to come first. For me, skincare doesn't need to involve scent – I tend to lean on perfume or cologne if an aromatic experience is what I'm looking for. Additionally, Skingredients are vegan and cruelty-free.

There are just seven Skingredients products (so far!), as well as our good friend the Cleanse Off Mitt, covering cleansing, moisturising day and night, serum and SPF, designed to assist in skin health and provide protection for the future. It's a neat little capsule collection for your skin, giving you the optimum formulation for the non-negotiable parts of your skin routine.

Think of the quintessential balanced dinner plate, including the right amounts of carbs, fats, vitamins and protein, the things that we all need to be our healthiest selves, regardless of age and gender. This translates to skincare too. Your Core 4 is what you need, day in, day out, for skin health. And, in the same way you change up your eating habits at times depending on what you need, there are certain skincare ingredients you may need to add more of (depending on dryness, oiliness, etc.) and that's where the Mix + Match element comes in to play.

The Core 4 includes the four products everyone should use every day (full details on pages 146–149), and covers the checklist of ingredients to help in skin health: PreProbiotic Cleanse, a prebiotic-probiotic complex cleanser, Skin Veg, a hydrating and anti-ageing pre-serum, Skin Protein, a vitamin A and vitamin C serum, and Skin Shield, a broad-spectrum mineral SPF.

Once these beauties have your key skin nutrition arranged, you can then branch out into our Mix + Match routine, adding in the active salicylic acid cleanser, Sally Cleanse, the lactic acid + PHA cleanser, A-HA Cleanse, and the ceramide moisturiser, Skin Good Fats, as needed. As a facialist, I've learned that many skin concerns can come and go, so having a 'toolkit' of skincare, with products you can lean on for more temporary concerns, is incredibly valuable. What you need can depend on age, nutrition, stress levels, menstrual cycle – any one of a number of factors can knock your skin out of sync. Mix + Match responds depending on what your skin needs.

Targeted skincare is, of course, all about the results and there are plenty of case studies on the website, showing the visible results experienced by users. Eighteen months prior to the launch, we began an initiative called Project Love Your Skin (See Skingredients on Instagram). We encouraged those who didn't feel confident in their skin to get in contact, and from there, we selected as many hoomans as we could to take part in a secret trial of Skingredients. The participants' testimonials and progress pictures are incredible and truly emotional to see. Improving your skin health may not change your entire life, but it can make a significant difference in how you carry yourself and how you feel. Results included – and still include – improved skin texture, less redness, plumper and smoother skin, less obvious pores, less noticeable pigment, i.e. blotchiness, improved healing ability, fewer spots appearing (and the spots that occur not leaving behind those dreaded post-inflammatory hyperpigmentation marks). But, ultimately, it is the messages that pour into Nerd HQ from hoomans who say their lives have changed, their confidence has grown ... that is the true reason behind this skincare range right there, in the emotional results.

Pump Action

It's not just the vibrant exterior design of Skingredients that we spent time perfecting, we also gave long and serious thought to the type of delivery system the bottle would have. After lots of discussion, we went with opaque, airless pump containers for the whole range. This is because some of the ingredients, particularly vitamins C and A, can be averse to light and oxygen. Those elements do not bring out the best in certain forms of vitamin C at all – they make it deteriorate pretty rapidly. The airless pump option gave us great delivery without destabilising the formulation. All the goodness is kept safe and stable inside, waiting in perfect condition to do its thing when you pump.

The Cleanse Off Mitt (COM)™

There's another product in the range that's as hardworking as all the rest: the Cleanse Off Mitt (COM) is a microfibre tool used prior to your cleanser and to remove cleanser for a thorough cleanse, or as a stand-alone to rival wipes. Prompted by my (well-documented) dislike of the facial wipe and the negative effects they can have on the skin, I devised a plan for an affordable and reusable alternative. The COM removes all makeup naturally – even mascara. For thorough cleansing, run it under water, wring it out, pop it on your hand and glide it across your face to remove makeup, oil and debris. The Cleanse Off Mitt is also your cleansing tool, allowing you to remove your cleanser without the typical puddles under your sink. You can do the Jesus Christ Test (see page 86) to check that it does all that – and I guarantee you will be pleasantly astounded.

For cleaning, you simply hand wash it with antibacterial soap and pop it in the machine at 30°C or lower once a week – because of this, we recommend having three on the go and replacing your mitts after three months of use for best results.

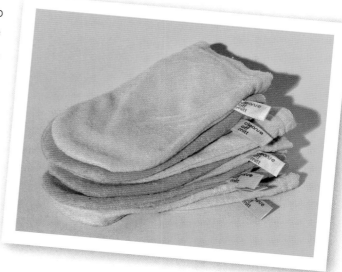

The skinny on Skingredients

Here they are: seven kickass formulations and one serious cleansing mitt. It's a small but perfectly formed range.

Skingredient	What it actively targets
Cleanse Off Mitt	The compact blue mitt that means business, gently and respectfully removing makeup, oil and debris with just water. This is your first step, A.M. and P.M., so that you can cleanse, serum, SPF and what have you with nothing in the way. It's suitable for all skin types, concerns, ages and genders – even super-sensitive skin.
The Core 4: 01 PreProbiotic Cleanse – hydrating and nourishing cleanser	This is all about the three Ps: prebiotics, probiotics and polyhydroxy acid (PHA). Prebiotics and probiotics work to soothe the skin and nurture your skin's balance. PreProbiotic cleanses, hydrates and gently exfoliates the skin for plumpness, softness and hydration. The formulation is feather-light, non-greasy, yet has the muscle to remove oil and makeup, including eye makeup. It's gentle enough that you can use it A.M. and P.M. It's non-comedogenic, meaning it doesn't clog pores, so it's suitable for the oily and congestion-prone as well. It's a comfort blanket for even the driest of dry skin because it's deeply nourishing. It can be used as a soothing micro-mask, too.
The Core 4: 02 Skin Veg – hydrating and brightening pre-serum	Skin Veg is your A.M. and P.M. skin superjuice of hyaluronic acid, PHA, a pro-collagen peptide, and fruit, veg and botanical extracts. It works to hydrate, brighten and protect your skin from the environmental factors that can cause it to age faster. It provides instant hydration and long-term anti-ageing, with broccoli extract, tomato extract and radish root extract. PHA (polyhydroxy acid, specifically gluconolactone) allows active ingredients to penetrate optimally to help your routine to work harder. It's ultra-lightweight and suitable for all skin types: oily, dry and sensitive and everything in between. I recommend you apply it post-cleansing and prior to other serums (or mixed in with other serums) for a shot of dewy plumpness.

Key active elements and why	Suitable for
Microfibre has a positive charge when water is added, so it works like a makeup and oil magnet. These polyester loops are superfine – same diameter as hair and break the surface tension between the oil on skin and oil in makeup, thus removing easily.	 eye makeup remover suitable for mamas-to-be 
Alpha-glucan oligosaccharide: a skin-soothing prebiotic. Lactobacillus: a dairy-free probiotic that boosts skin's natural moisturising factor for hydrated skin. Gluconolactone: a PHA for hydration and ultra-mild yet effective exfoliation.	 eye makeup remover suitable for mamas-to-be 
Clinically proven pro-collagen peptide: a peptide is a chain of amino acids that works to signal to the skin to do something – in this case, to create more collagen, which allows lines and wrinkles to appear reduced. Sodium hyaluronate: low molecular weight hyaluronic acid to hydrate the skin deeply. Gluconolactone: a polyhydroxy acid that assists in product absorption. Fruit and veg extracts: soothing, nourishing and antioxidant. Liquorice root extract: a botanical brightening ingredient and antioxidant.	 suitable for use around the eye suitable for mamas-to-be 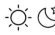

Skingredient	What it actively targets
The Core 4: 03 Skin Protein – anti-ageing vitamin A and C serum	Skin Protein is your results-driven vitamin A serum to smooth, tighten and brighten. Retinyl palmitate is a form of vitamin A that you are now well aware of, having read this far! With added vitamin C for antioxidant protection and that phenomenal pro-collagen peptide clinically proven to reduce the appearance of lines and wrinkles, Skin Protein is designed to be used both A.M. and P.M. It also contains good fats in the form of sunflower seed oil to hydrate and soothe the skin. Formulated for all skin types, it addresses a wide range of skin concerns, including dullness, lines and wrinkles, lax skin, dark circles, blackheads, whiteheads, lumps, bumps, large pores and excessive oiliness. Not suitable for use during pregnancy.
The Core 4: 04 Skin Shield SPF 50 PA +++ – broad-spectrum light protection	Skin Shield SPF is a priming and moisturising broad-spectrum mineral SPF lotion that protects your skin from sunlight as well as blue light from screens and pollution daily. It's like an invisible parasol, protecting you from UVA rays, UVB rays, pollution and HEV light (blue light, the light emitted from screens). It has a peachy tint so there's no need to stress about a chalky white cast or photo flashback. It's non-comedogenic, oil-free, water-resistant and non-greasy. A superstar, in other words! It's suitable for all skin types, and has a dewy finish for a natural skin-like glow.
Mix + Match: A-HA Cleanse – Lactic acid treatment cleanser + resurfacing micro-mask *Returning to shelves in 2021*	A-HA Cleanse is an 8 per cent lactic acid and 2 per cent polyhydroxy acid cleanser that cleanses, exfoliates and brightens, and works to boost your skin's natural moisturising factor (NMF) to help improve skin hydration. Formulated to bring about brighter, more even, smoother and better hydrated skin, A-HA Cleanse can be used as a treatment cleanser every second night for extra va-va-voom. It does away with the need for a toner and is your non-grit, no-scrubs exfoliator for more even skin.

Key active elements and why	Suitable for
Vitamin A (retinyl palmitate): an ester form of vitamin A and retinol alternative that speeds up skin cell renewal and re-educates the skin in a gentler approach. Beta carotene: a precursor to vitamin A with antioxidant benefits, it triggers vitamin A within the skin. Clinically proven pro-collagen peptide: reduces the depth and appearance of lines and wrinkles. Vitamin C (ascorbic acid + ascorbyl palmitate) and vitamin E: potent antioxidants. Rooibos tea extract + green tea extract: more potent antioxidants. Sunflower seed oil: hydrating, ingredient rich in fatty acids	 **suitable for use around the eye** **not suitable for pregnant hoomans™** 
Zinc oxide: a mineral that works as a physical SPF filter (SPF 50, PA +++). Niacinamide (vitamin B3): an antioxidant that can improve skin tone and texture. Vitamin E: a potent antioxidant to protect from free-radical damage. Allantoin: a moisturising ingredient that smooths the skin.	 **suitable for use around the eye** **suitable for mamas-to-be**
Lactic acid: hydrating alpha-hydroxy acid (AHA) that encourages the skin's own exfoliation, has a larger molecule so is better suited to more sensitive skin. Polyhydroxy acid: a mild exfoliating form of an AHA, with an even larger molecule.	 **not suitable for eye make up removal** **suitable for mamas-to-be** Not suitable for daily use – should be used every third evening (not mornings)

Skingredient	What it actively targets
Mix + Match: Sally Cleanse – salicylic acid active cleanser, spot-zapper and micro-mask	Sally Cleanse is an active cleanser with 2 per cent salicylic acid, which is the highest amount of salicylic acid permitted in cosmetics in the EU. This hero cleanser helps to clear pores and reduce congestion such as lumps, bumps, whiteheads and blackheads, while encouraging the skin to exfoliate itself. As Sally is an active product, it's designed to be used every third night alongside 01 PreProbiotic Cleanse. It's a potent cleanser that must be handled with care and expert guidance. It is specifically formulated for skin – face or body – with excess oil, blackheads, whiteheads and lumps and bumps in any form. It does away with the need for a separate toner and cleanser because it has both angles covered. Also serves as a wash-off spot-zapper and as a micro-mask.
Mix + Match: Skin Good Fats – moisturising ceramide balm	Skin Good Fats is your not-so-typical moisturiser. Our chubby little moisturising balm contains the same fats that make up your skin's barrier, including ceramide NP, to deeply hydrate, and a clinically proven, patented anti-irritation ingredient to stop those itches. It is an occlusive top layer for those who love the feeling of a moisturiser and those with dry or irritated skin that needs some loving and healing.

Key active elements and why	Suitable for
Salicylic acid: a beta hydroxy acid (BHA) that dissolves oil and debris in the pores and exfoliates the skin.	not suitable for eye make up removal not suitable for pregnant hoomans™ Not suitable for daily use – should be used every third evening (not mornings)
Ceramide NP: a skin-native lipid known to help improve skin barrier function. Shea butter glycerides: a moisturising ingredient derived from shea butter fatty acids. Avena sativa (oat) kernel extract: a clinically proven anti-irritant with antihistamine properties. Vitis vinifera (grape) seed oil: a moisturising oil with antioxidant properties. Niacinamide (vitamin B3) and vitamin E: potent antioxidants to fight free-radical damage.	suitable for use around the eye suitable for mamas-to-be

Why is Sally a Rock Star?

Salicylic acid is an active ingredient and as such it is governed by strict regulations. In the EU, this means that 2 per cent is the maximum amount of salicylic acid allowed in any cosmetic retail product. Our Sally is beloved because it combats oiliness and congestion by dissolving the dead skin plugs in the pores. It can do this because it is oil soluble, therefore can cut through the sebum your skin naturally produces or, at times, overproduces. If you're facing a breakout, Sally is your best friend and ally. It can penetrate through the stratum corneum (the outer layer of your skin), which is the layer that locks in moisture and keeps irritants out. Once in there, Sally works to exfoliate the skin by getting into the pores and dissolving them of blockages, whether these occur in the form of excess oil, dead skin cells, makeup residue or pollution. It is brilliant for keratosis pilaris too (chicken skin; see page 92) on the body. Its anti-inflammatory properties mean it will work on soothing redness and irritation at the same time, making it an excellent weapon in your battle against flare-ups. The beauty of salicylic acid is that it is robust and effective, which means you don't have to exfoliate the life out of your skin to get the results you want. For skin-respectful (gentler than scrubs) but determined exfoliation that nurtures the skin, Sally is just the ticket. But even though Sally can be gentler, it's still incredibly important to follow directions when it comes to chemical exfoliation, as you can still overuse or misuse it. Less is more – remove Sally Cleanse thoroughly and don't overuse.

Find out more with the hashtag #Skingredients on Instagram, or follow us at @skingredients. We look forward to chatting!

Chapter 8

Conscious Skincare

Is it possible to choose 100 per cent sustainable skincare? This is a huge question and the answer isn't straightforward or simple. It's brilliant and heartening to know that a lot of consumers today want to make eco-friendly, ethical choices and embrace conscious consumerism – rightfully so, as we all have a responsibility to the world. I'm in exactly the same position – I want to play my part in protecting the environment through my spending choices, and as a creator of products I am also, if not even more so, uber-conscious of trying to make our own processes and products more sustainable. But at this moment in time, in 2020, is it really possible to make 100 per cent sustainable, ethical skincare choices? I'm afraid not. That time is coming, but there is a whole spectrum of change required to achieve this, criss-crossing a number of industries, so consumers have to be patient until the skindustry gets all its ducks in a row.

Sustainable skincare

There is no single definition for the term 'sustainable' that everyone can agree on. For some people, the primary concern is about recycled and recyclable packaging; for others it's having an ethical supply chain, carbon-neutral distribution methods or sustainable ingredients that aren't causing a ripple effect in nature. When you pick a bottle from the shelf, there are lots of component parts that go into it being there. Some can be controlled by the product maker, some can't. It's very frustrating as it's not clear-cut, but the good news is that progress is being made. The even better news is that you have considerable purchase power – supply will always strive to meet demand, so you make your demands heard through your choices and that will keep fuelling those all-important changes across the board.

What do you look for in sustainable skincare?

Holly White, vegan cookbook author and lifestyle blogger at Holly.ie, fully behind the purchase power movement, answers:

I always felt that the loudest voice you will ever have is how and where you spend your money, so I am conscious to support brands that share my values. I look for utmost transparency with regard to animal testing and ingredients. Sustainably sourced organic ingredients support communities and ensure that the land can regenerate year after year, so buying from companies that are using organic components is a great way to support Mother Nature. I think social media has made it easier to see brands' key values. And I'm interested in what charities a brand might support or what causes they care about.

Lastly, when a product is finished, I always want to be able to recycle or compost packaging so that's an important factor to consider. It's not always possible, but I do think more brands are moving that way by removing unnecessary inserts and spatulas and streamlining things.

You know by now that I like honesty, which is why I didn't call this chapter 'Sustainable Skincare' because I don't think we can quite promise that yet 100 per cent. I think it's essential to be well informed and to make the very best skincare choices you can, for your skin and for the environment, but I understand that as an individual there's only so much you can do to support sustainability right now, so remain conscious but do not place too much pressure on yourself – skincare is an interlinked industry, which is why it takes brands time to fully switch to sustainable methods the whole way through the production process. Critics say the industry is too slow-moving in this regard, but progress here is dependent on other partners – packagers, etc – to update their processes to sustainable ones, which takes time. This is particularly the case for small brands operating with limited resources in a highly competitive market. Significant change requires a cross-chain revamp of thinking with regard to methods. Yes, you can support this by demanding it, and I hope you do, but it's going to take time to get us all there.

All brands are aware of the need for change by now, so they should all be working on it, but some are further down the road than others. We all have a part to play in making wiser decisions daily and, ultimately, align ourselves with brands taking this as seriously as it deserves.

We at The Skin Nerd are committed to doing what we can to make our products more sustainable by 2021. As part of this effort, we have signed up to the Repak Members' Plastic Pledge, which commits us to reducing plastic packaging waste in order to meet the goals set out in the EU Circular Economy Package. Initiatives like this provide excellent guidance and incentives to businesses to do better – and we will!

So, what can you do? You can be aware of the options, what to look out for and the values of each brand you're purchasing. To help you do your best to make conscious skincare choices, I've listed below the elements to consider.

Least sustainable choices

* Non-recycled packaging
* Non-recyclable packaging
* Ingredients that are not sustainably sourced
* Processes that don't take the environment into consideration (seek out brands that provide information about their sustainable processes)
* Not cruelty-free
* Non-vegan

Mid-level sustainable choices

* Recyclable packaging
* Facilitates recycling on your behalf
* Sustainably sourced ingredients
* Reduced packaging
* Use of renewable energy formats
* Use of renewable ingredients
* International transit kept to a minimum throughout the production process

Very sustainable choices

* Glass containers
* Refillable containers
* Recycled packaging
* Locally sourced ingredients
* Ethically sourced ingredients
* Locally packaged (EU or UK)

Nerdie note: if a brand has one very sustainable element but doesn't work on everything else, this does not make it better than a brand that ticks all the boxes of the mid-level sustainable list. And decisions regarding sustainability aren't always straightforward – a company may want to source packaging made locally in order to reduce their carbon footprint when it comes to transport but this packaging may not be recyclable. And that can make your decision-making process as a consumer harder too.

Unfortunately, very sustainable skincare may be more expensive for the consumer because the brand is paying more money for each stage in its production process due to use of optimum ingredients, packaging and distribution channels. So that is hard for all involved but is slowly changing for the better all the time as sustainable slowly becomes the norm. You might feel frustrated by the choices currently available to you and perhaps priced out of doing the right thing, but take heart from the fact that it will change over the coming years and the cost of your sustainable choices should come down to a more purse-friendly level.

The Skin Nerd recommends

If you want to choose sustainable options, there are plenty of brands making good strides in this area. Their efforts are very impressive and becoming more so all the time as they figure out how exactly to get all the elements humming together in a sustainable chorus. For my money, I can recommend these pioneering beauties:

REN
REN is on a mission to make their range as sustainable as possible and to that end have introduced 'infinity plastic' packaging – recycled plastic that can go on to be recycled again.

Dr Hauschka
This brand uses plant-based formulations, biodynamic farming methods to grow their ingredients and green electricity to fuel this.

Evolve Beauty
This Hertfordshire-based, small-batch skincare brand uses recyclable

packaging. Their PET plastic bottles are 75 per cent recycled plastic and are themselves recyclable. They source ingredients as close to them locally as possible, and ensure they are fair trade and sustainable sources. Their products contain intriguing bioactives like coconut peptides, so definitely worth a shout for the active ingredient lover who craves sustainability.

L'Occitane

This Provence-inspired brand is focused on reducing the use of plastic, with a commitment to have 100 per cent recycled bottles that are also recyclable within the next five years.

The Body Shop

The grandmother of sustainable skincare! Committed to ethical trading, recycling and working for the improvement of the communities that harvest their ingredients.

Aveda

American company Aveda uses ethically sourced ingredients and has a commitment to improving the communities in India, Nepal, Madagascar and Ethiopia that grow its ingredients. It is also focused on creating eco-friendly packaging through the use of post-consumer recycled (PCR) materials. The entire product line will be vegan within two years.

Clarins

This brand is a committed member of the Plastic Odyssey challenge to collect plastic waste from the oceans, is focused on recyclable packaging and its HQ in Paris is home to 160,000 bees that thrive in its roof-top hives!

UpCircle

This UK-based brand was originally created as a way to use old coffee grounds – now, they have a range of products that are all 100 per cent vegan, cruelty-free, sustainable and use repurposed ingredients, and their packaging is fully recyclable.

Medik8

As it's both a to-professional and a to-consumer brand, it is a bit harder for Medik8. Nonetheless, their glass packaging is made of 40 per cent recycled glass (in turn easily recycled), and their professional products are made of 100 per cent recycled materials that can be recycled.

I'm very happy to be able to say that the **Irish sustainability pioneers** are more than holding their own and doing their bit brilliantly:

Nunaïa

With recyclable glass bottles, recyclable paper and cardboard packaging and sustainability-oriented supply chains, as well as an Ecocert COSMOS ORGANIC certification and a Vegan Society certification, Nunaïa nourishes the skin with bioactive formulations inspired by nature.

Codex Beauty Bia Collection

Filled with bioactives that soothe and protect the skin, Codex Beauty products are housed in packaging made from sugarcane ethanol and have an Ecocert COSMOS ORGANIC certification.

The Burren Perfumery

Inspired by the beautiful Burren landscape in County Clare, this brand produces organic cosmetics and perfumes focusing on quality over quantity, in addition to natural skincare with calming essential oils. Their soaps are wrapped in FSC sustainable paper (from responsibly managed forests), and their plastic bottles are made of 100 per cent post-consumer recycled plastic. They're truly ethical and passion-driven – a beauty to see and a beauty to use!

Human+Kind

Founded in Cork, Human+Kind uses sustainably sourced ingredients in their products.

Ethical skincare

You'll often hear the words 'sustainable' and 'ethical' bandied about as if they are interchangeable, but they mean different things. Sustainable, as we've seen, is about the processes behind the product, whereas ethical skincare means that the formulation inside the bottle is:

* cruelty-free
* vegan
* natural (as explained on page 105)
* organic.

Cruelty-free

As may seem obvious, this means that the product has not been tested on animals at any point during its design and production. The EU has had a strict law in place since 2013 banning the sale of personal care products tested on animals. While this is reassuring for consumers, the EU law does not extend to companies' activities in other markets, so while your European skincare product might not be animal tested, the company that produced it might do animal testing on products sold outside the EU. Your best defence against this possibility is to make like Alice in Wonderland and follow the rabbit – in this case, the Leaping Bunny logo. This tells you that the company's core value is to be cruelty-free and it doesn't conduct animal tests anywhere in the world. Products can be cruelty-free without having the Leaping Bunny certification. Another popular cruelty-free certification is the PETA Beauty Without Bunnies certification.

Vegan

This means that the product contains no animal or animal-derived ingredients. It usually translates into an ingredients list composed of plants, minerals and safe synthetic ingredients. The Vegan Society provides accreditation for skincare products that meet the requirements; if they pass, they can display their logo.

Again, as with cruelty-free, a brand and its products can be vegan-friendly without having the certification.

Organic

Organic products are often plant-based and the ingredients are farmed using sustainable and chemical-free methods (free from pesticides). But there is no regulation at present regarding the use of the term 'organic' in the EU which means that less dedicated brands could use a bit of organic stuff and then slap 'Organic' on the label. However, the words 'Certified Organic' on the label indicate that 95 per cent of the ingredients are indeed organic. If the packaging uses the words 'Made with organic ingredients', you're possibly looking at an organic ingredient component of less than 70 per cent.

The Ecocert COSMOS ORGANIC certification means that a brand does not use GMOs (genetically modified organisms) in their ingredients, uses

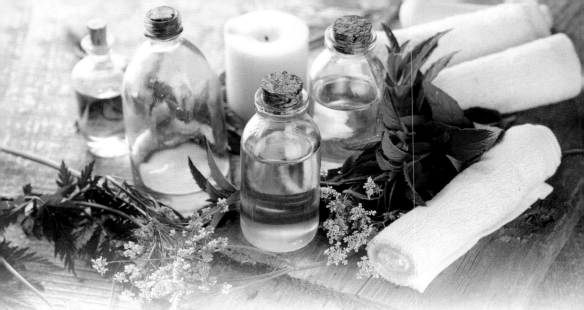

natural resources responsibly, respects biodiversity, has environmentally friendly production, uses no petrochemical ingredients and uses recyclable packaging. If 95 per cent of the plants within a product are organic, it can be certified COSMOS ORGANIC.

The Seventh Nerdie Principle

Be kind. Yep, it's another solid but simple principle by which we live at Nerd HQ. I am all for kindness in the everyday, random acts of kindness, the deliberate acts of kindness, the impressive acts of kindness or the absent-minded acts of kindness … I'll take it whichever way you're offering it. In skincare, this means lots of things:

- Be kind to your less-than-perfect skin – it's just doing its best.
- Be kind to your gut with a healthy diet, because that will help your skin hugely.
- Be kind to your body with good lifestyle choices.

- Be kind to the environment by choosing sustainable products where you can.
- Be kind to your fellow hoomans by choosing ethical products.
- Be kind to the future generations by making the best consumer choices you can with informed purchase power.

You'll be wrecked from all that kindness! And when you are, do yourself the kindness of a good pre-bed skin routine for a good night's sleep.

PROTOCOL:

Conscious skincare at home

- **Minimal purchasing:** Less and better is the way to go when buying skincare products. Do your research, figure out what you feel you need, invest in a consultation to get expert input and then buy small amounts of excellent formulations. And the good ones tend to require you to apply far less to the skin. You just need to be skin-thrifty!
- **Double up:** Make each product work as hard as possible with dual function. For example, buy an eye-safe serum rather than a separate eye cream.
- **Do a shelf audit:** Root out every bit of makeup and skincare from every hiding place and put it all on the table to see what you have. (Also a good opportunity to check use-by dates!) Perhaps there's stuff you've forgotten and would absolutely love to use? Or

maybe it was forgotten for a reason because it was a wine o'clock online purchase that really isn't you? In that case, can you swap with a friend and get something you'd use from her stash? Can you regift it? Donate it? Make sure you maintain a sensible range that features only those products you love and that love your skin – a toolkit of the ingredients you need for days where your skin is more dehydrated, more red, days when you have spots – anything beyond this that you don't use can be swapped or charity shopped (make sure your charity shop accepts skincare, and find out if it needs to be unopened or not). Be a discerning diva, in other words – the Earth will thank you for it!

- **Treat your tools right:** If you keep your skincare accessories in good nick, such as your brushes, Cleanse Off Mitt, and your electricals if you are a skin-tech fanatic, they will perform better, for longer. It's simple skin maths!
- **Vampire those creams:** This means lids on and kept out of direct sunlight. The formulations inside your gorgeous bottles can degrade in direct sunlight, so ensure their optimum performance and endurance by storing them correctly – locked tight in the shadows.
- **Make at-home recycling easier:** Put a recycling bin in the bathroom so you're more likely to bin all those consciously bought recyclable packages correctly.

Part Two Skin Takeaways

1. **Know *your* Rock Star Ingredients** and make them part of your daily routine. This is easily done via a skin consultation, but if you don't want to go that route, then assess your skin status in the mirror and your desired skin results, then go back over these chapters and (taking your age into account) match up those with the abilities of the ingredients as described here. Note the details in your Personal Action Plan.

2. When you have identified the right ingredients and products for you, **apply them consistently**. There are no holidays in skincare, no 'I forgot', no 'the dog ate my SPF' – it's *daily* skincare, no excuses! If you're not consistent, you won't feel the benefits.

3. Remember that **proper skin health requires a holistic approach**. You can't just lash on a pile of vitamin A and think, 'that's me done'. There's no single solution – there are only interconnected solutions. That's why I talk about skincare, gut health, exercise and stress with equal emphasis. They all play an active role in your skin status and skin health, so it's in your best interest to take the big-picture view.

4. It's important to exercise your **purchase power** to influence how products are made and sold.

5. **Practise conscious consumerism** regarding your skincare choices because that will force/encourage the skindustry to tick all of the sustainable and ethical boxes, which will be to the benefit of all people, everywhere.

6 Do everything you can to ensure that you are making **educated and informed skincare choices**. I know your budget might put certain constraints on you – let's face it, that goes for all of us – but you can always find good products in your price bracket. Remember to research, buy less and buy better – that way, you won't feel the pinch of the cost so much. I'm tempted to say you're worth it, but, you know …

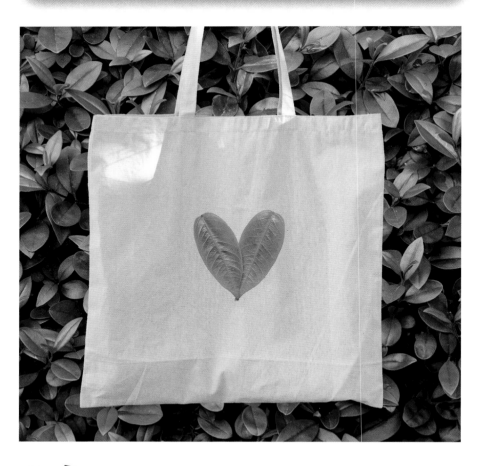

THE SKIN NERD PHILOSOPHY

3

What You Need to Do: From Skincare Routines to Treatments and Expert Guidance

The gloves are on!

This is where you get to have fun and do all the things you've learned in Parts 1 and 2. So far, we have looked at the thinking behind skincare, giving you all the knowledge you need to make good choices for your skin. Now we'll look at skincare routines and what you can do for your skin, both at home and at a clinic or salon.

Proactive, positive skincare choices don't necessarily have to depend on lots of money and time – you can tailor a routine to fit your clock and pocket. And to prove it to you, I've set out a number of different routines, starting with a 30-second per day routine. There is no way you can look me in the eye and tell me you can't manage to fence off half a minute in your day to take care of yourself! I've also included case studies of real-life skin scenarios and how to handle them, so that you can find your best fit and start implementing your very own unique routine, one that suits you. You'll come away with a different idea about what you can and can't do, I promise.

When it comes to skincare, as you know by now, I have always been an advocate of the 360° approach. I also talk a lot about the fact that so many different elements and people can play a role in our skincare approach – department store skincare counters, active ingredients, facialists, consultants, pharmacies, GPs, herbalists, dermatologists – and that we all need to work as one in order to be able to help and advise those who need it. It is, in my opinion, unethical to give skincare

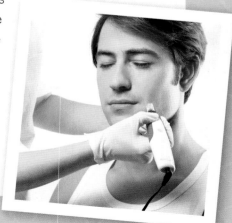

advice to a person with a skin condition, such as cystic acne or psoriasis, without referring them to a medical professional. A good skincare consultant will advise alongside a GP or dermatologist to ensure that daily skincare routines are working at optimum level.

Similarly, if stress is an underlying issue when it comes to the skin, a holistic approach is required in order to equip the hooman with the tools they can use to tackle that stress is required. There's no point simply giving that person a balm to calm the skin irritation when they would also clearly benefit from the advice of a mental health professional regarding stress-management techniques that will have a positive impact on their mind and body health, and in turn positively affect their skin.

I always aim to work in tandem with my fellow professionals, to provide a complementary service that uses the expertise of the whole sector. I put optimum skin health at the centre of everything I do, and the client and I reach this by whatever means best suit their particular situation. With this in mind, I have compiled for you a unique skin expert jigsaw puzzle – the key is that no single piece completes the set, all must be present and fit together to ensure a comprehensive approach to skincare.

As part of this, I have rounded up insights from a group of skincare professionals whose work interlinks in this way to help you better understand this multi-disciplinary approach. I've spoken with a GP, a skin therapist, a dietitian, a dermatologist, a cosmetic doctor, a plastic surgeon, a pharmacist, a psychodermatologist and a fitness expert and each of them will explain how they work within the skin professional jigsaw puzzle, showing you what expertise is available, advising you on when you should seek their help and explaining which of them is your best choice for your skin query or issue.

Chapter 9

Your 'Everything Skin' Protocols

We have aced the theory, now it's time to get down to some hands-on work. This chapter is about implementing a nurturing daily skincare routine. We'll break it down into the fundamental parts, then explain some routines that can fit into even the busiest of busy days which will enable you to topically treat your skin for optimum health and clarity.

The daily skincare non-negotiables

Our essential 360° approach to skincare (though I'm sure you don't need reminding by now) means nutrition and possibly supplements on the inside, active and cosmetic skincare on the outside, and SPF and mineral makeup on top. When I talk about a daily skincare routine, I'm focusing on the basics needed to maintain your skin's health and encourage even better health. And you'll be happy to hear that the basics, the non-negotiables, the daily must-dos are three easy-peasy steps.

Step 1. Cleanser

It's not a nice thought, but our skin has lots of uninvited guests vying to take up residence on it every day – air pollution, bacteria, grime – and our skin does the valiant work of keeping all this daily debris at bay, but it needs our help in dealing with it. I am a staunch believer in daily cleansing – even if beauty trends come along every now and then that suggest otherwise. Nothing anyone says can convince me that daily cleansing is not a spectacularly good idea and a key part of establishing the right foundation for skin health.

In fact, I am devoted to the double cleanse. 'Double the work!', I hear you cry. 'Double the cleanliness!' I shout right back. And double the results! Yes, it does take more time – but we're talking seconds here. 120 seconds, to be precise.

So, how to perform a good double cleanse? First, remove your makeup – *not* with a facial wipe (shudder). This is your pre-cleanse phase, removing makeup, oils, debris and SPF on the skin's surface and prepping your skin for the main event. My preference for a thorough pre-cleanse is my own Cleanse Off Mitt (COM), which does the job beautifully with just water added, mechanically removing the majority of makeup. Alternatively, I adore an oil or cleansing balm such as Dermalogica PreCleanse Balm or Nunaïa Superfood Cleansing Balm with the COM for heavy-duty makeup days. Next, use a cleanser that will soothe, nourish or treat your skin. The cleansers that nourish and soothe usually don't contain active ingredients – their function is to pacify the skin and help to balance it – whereas an active cleanser, as we've covered, will target skin issues. An active cleanser is a treatment, every few nights, and is usually an exfoliating product.

Passive cleanser recommendations

* Avène Extremely Gentle Cleansing Lotion is a great product for the very sensitive skinned, or for those who are experiencing skin irritation. This cleanser works gently and does not irritate the skin even if literally everything else does.

- Probiotic cleansers like those from Biofresh (a cleansing milk, best for dry/dehydrated/mature skins) or Gallinée (a probiotic foaming wash perfect for oilier, normal skin types or people who prefer a wash to a milk or a creamy cleanser) as they are mild yet still help to balance the skin.

- Skingredients PreProbiotic Cleanse contains a prebiotic-probiotic complex plus PHA for skin calmness and hydration.

- Kiehl's Midnight Recovery Botanical Cleansing Oil is a lightweight oil-to-milk cleanser particularly effective for dehydrated or dry skin, or as a pre-cleanser for those with oilier skin.

- IMAGE Ormedic Balancing Cleanser is a wash cleanser best for normal to combination or oily skin containing soothing, antioxidant green tea and aloe vera with hydrating hyaluronic acid, and can be used A.M. and P.M.

- ASAP Gentle Eye Makeup Remover is great for thoroughly removing eye makeup remover without damaging lash extensions (which I'm very fond of).

Active cleanser recommendations

For exfoliation, oiliness and decongestion:
- IMAGE Clear Cell Clarifying Cleanser contains salicylic acid (rock star alert), IMAGE granactive acne complex, arnica for inflammation and tea tree.

- Environ Clarity+ Sebu-Wash Gel Cleanser contains a mild amount of salicylic acid, hydrating glycerin and tea tree. Ideal for teen skin and Environ also state that it is suitable for use during pregnancy.

- Skingredients Sally Cleanse contains 2 per cent salicylic acid, so Sally ain't one to be messed with and should be used once every three nights and no more.

For exfoliation and dullness:
- IMAGE Ageless Total Facial Cleanser includes glycolic acid plus green tea extract so this baby keeps your skin bright and balanced.

- Neostrata Foaming Glycolic Wash contains a whopping 18 per cent glycolic acid plus 2 per cent PHA (lactobionic acid) which come together to exfoliate.

Great for those with pigmentation, those looking to tackle fine lines and wrinkles, those with mild congestion and advanced glycolic acid users.

* Kate Somerville ExfoliKate Daily Foaming Cleanser contains glycolic acid, lactic acid and enzymes for gentle yet effective exfoliation.
* Skingredients A-HA Cleanse contains 8 per cent lactic acid with 2 per cent polyhydroxy acid for a gentle exfoliation and a thorough cleanse.

Toners

As I've mentioned already, toners can be a useful way of getting additional key ingredients onto your skin, i.e. peptides, exfoliating acids or hydrators, but in my opinion they aren't an essential, and should not be on your list if you're looking to build a solid skincare routine for the first time and are trying to keep to a tight budget.

The type of toners I disapprove of are those that work *only* to remove oils from the skin and keep it mattified. Don't get me wrong, on occasion I want matte skin just as much as the next hooman, but my problem is with how toners go about it: often, they're high in drying alcohols or super astringent ingredients that will dehydrate the skin and even impair its barrier. Not worth it, in my opinion. Hydrating spritzes or toners serve a different function though and I highly approve of spritzing (more on this shortly).

Step 2. Serum

It might be a controversial statement, but for my money a good serum can work far better than a moisturiser when it comes to results beyond hydration. A serum tends to have smaller molecules and a thinner consistency than most moisturisers so it can get down into the skin and hydrate at a deeper level, as well as providing the skin with the nutrition it needs to create its own hydration. Due to their thickness, moisturisers sit on top of the skin and condition the uppermost layers rather than hydrate deeper down. So, for me, step two is always a serum because not only does it deliver a really good blast of hydration, it truly penetrates and targets the skin cells, which a moisturiser cannot do as its purpose is to moisturise at a superficial level.

If you don't already have a serum as part of your skincare routine, then I recommend you start with a vitamin A one. Vitamin A is a stellar all-rounder for skin concerns and general skin health. In the form of retinyl palmitate, it can help to repair the cells within the skin and promote their general health, which means that many skin concerns are tackled in one go, including pigmentation (sun spots, discolouration, etc.), fine lines, dullness, lax skin and more. You can also double up a vitamin A serum as a moisturiser, anti-ager and hydrator for the eye area (checking first that it's safe for this use), so no need for a separate eye product. Please note that vitamin A products are not recommended during pregnancy and some people may have sensitivity to harder-hitting retinol products. Where your main serum will help to improve the general health of your skin to help tackle your concerns, a secondary serum will include ingredients that work towards your particular issue – for example, brightening ingredients if you are tackling pigmentation, more hydrators if you have very dry skin, peptides and perhaps an acid if you are targeting the signs of ageing.

Serums can target specific concerns, which is one of their great benefits. Here is a brief list of the four key skin needs/concerns and some of the serums that can achieve them.

Brightening	Hydrating	Reducing Redness	Anti-Ageing
Skingredients Skin Veg	Skingredients Skin Good Fats	DMK Beta Gel	IMAGE Vital C Hydrating Antioxidant ACE Serum
IMAGE Iluma Intense Brightening Serum	Codex Skin Superfood	Environ Focus Care Colostrum Gel	Environ Skin EssentiA AVST Moisturiser

Brightening	Hydrating	Reducing Redness	Anti-Ageing
Murad Rapid Age Spot Corrector	IMAGE Ageless Total Pure Hyaluronic Filler	Neostrata Restore Redness Neutralizing Serum	Skingredients Skin Protein
Alpha-H Vitamin B	MRL Skin Quencher	Dr. Jart+ Cicapair Tiger Grass Serum	Dr Dennis Gross C + Collagen Brighten + Firm Vitamin C Serum

Step 3. SPF/Sunscreen

SPF isn't glamorous or instantly transformative, but it is an essential. We've already covered SPF in detail in Chapter 5, so here I'll just give you the lowdown on reading the label and my recommended products.

The sun's UVB rays are the rays mainly responsible for reddening and burning the skin, and they are also a culprit in the development of melanoma. The SPF number on the bottle informs you of the level of UVB protection within the product.

So what does your SPF do against these damaging rays?

* SPF 50 protects against 98% of UVB rays
* SPF 30 protects against 97% of UVB rays

You might be thinking, '1% difference, sure that's nothing, it doesn't matter which I use.' But wait! Look at it this way, maths nerd: SPF 50 allows 2% and SPF 30 allows 3%. So that means SPF 30 exposes you to 50 per cent more UV rays than SPF 50. Think of that next time you're choosing any SPF – for face or body. Another way of looking at it is that SPF 50 means it takes 50 times longer for the sun to get its fiery mitts on your skin than it would if you were wearing zero sun protection. (Again, much better than 30.)

The sun's UVA rays can penetrate glass and clouds and, as we've covered, they're also found in the blue light emitted from our electronic devices – which is why I'm forever telling you to wear SPF all the time, everywhere.

UVA protection has a few different modes of measurement that you'll see on packaging. The most common is probably the PA system, created in Japan – PA+ means that the product provides some UVA protection, PA++ means that it provides middling UVA protection, PA+++ means that it provides high UVA protection, and PA++++ means that it provides very high UVA protection.

SPF recommendations:
* Skingredients Skin Shield SPF 50 PA+++ – a mineral SPF with UVA, UVB, HEV, pollution and infrared protection, it's lightweight with no photo flashback (no white glow in photos due to a reflection caused by an SPF product) and a dewy finish.
* IMAGE Prevention+ Daily Matte Moisturiser SPF 32 – a mattifying long-lasting UVA and UVB protective daily moisturiser.
* Avène Tinted Mineral Fluid SPF 50+ – another mineral SPF with UVA and UVB protection, at a very accessible price point.
* For body SPF protection, I'd recommend Heliocare and Lancaster – because we can't just take care of our faces and forget the rest!
* For children, I'd recommend Avène and MooGoo.

That's it – your daily must-dos in a neat little nutshell (but I have included more detailed routines in this chapter too). Hopefully it's pretty clear to you now that you *do* have a time for daily routine. It's easy, especially once you get into the rhythm of it, a calming few minutes when you're not worrying about world events and instead think only about uncapping and applying. The balm of simplicity!

So, to recap on your daily routine, to be done morning and night:
The basic version:

1 Cleanse

2 Serum

3 SPF (A.M. only)

And the upgraded version:

1 Pre-cleanse

2 Cleanse

3 Active cleanse (these should only be used every 2–3 nights, as directed)

4 Serum

5 Secondary serum to target a specific concern

6 SPF (A.M. only)

Two serums should be sufficient, therefore no need for night moisturiser unless you like the feel of a barrier cream at night or if both serums are sticky and tacky – we understand the hooman desire to feel good.

Your next steps:

I'll be very happy to hear that you are doing a decent cleanse, applying a boosting serum and using SPF. That's a huge step towards excellent skin health. As you get the hang of it you can include what we consider the next essential steps: antioxidant protection and exfoliation.

Antioxidant products

You should get antioxidants into and onto your skin every day. You can eat them easily enough (see page 42). When it comes to skincare, you can apply antioxidant-enriched SPF/sunscreen and serums. Antioxidants are an unsung skincare hero, in my opinion, creating long-term protection. They are a clever investment in your skin because they fight free radicals and the damage they cause, protecting you from accelerated ageing. With antioxidants, the more of them in your routine, the better. This isn't an additional step but rather something to keep in mind when choosing serums and SPF.

Antioxidant recommendations

* Niod Survival 0
* Ultraceuticals Ultra Protective Antioxidant Complex
* Avène A-Oxitive Defense Serum
* Skingredients Skin Veg
* Neostrata SPFs such as their Sheer Physical SPF or Skin Matrix SPF

Exfoliation

Our skin should self-exfoliate as it did when we were kids but as we age, the skin cell turnover cycle slows down. Exfoliation is important because it allows us to decongest the pores, shed the dead cells that will steal our glow, and help the skin to operate at its best. You look fresher, younger and brighter, and products applied thereafter will be absorbed by the skin better. But we can obsess over exfoliating because it provides short-term gains. The problem with some (over-the-counter) products is that they can either be largely ineffective or way too abrasive – you either don't notice a single difference and feel hard done by, or it's so coarse you irritate the stratum corneum (the skin's outermost layer) which can lead to a compromised skin barrier.

Exfoliating with a non-abrasive cleanser that uses exfoliating acids or enzymes allows a more controlled mode of exfoliation that prompts your skin to exfoliate itself, and dissolves the bonds keeping a build-up of dead skin cells attached to the surface of the skin. In this respect, chemical (acid) exfoliation can be gentle when used correctly. The other bonus is that it won't require any forms of mechanical exfoliation, such as facial brushes or exfoliating pads. This is important because many experts say mechanical exfoliation can cause tiny tears on the surface of the skin. We would usually recommend and retail a targeted, active cleanser that does all the exfoliating for you.

Using an exfoliating cleanser every second to third night is recommended as it is an active treatment. Some skin concerns may need a bit more, but I don't recommend exfoliating more often than this without the help of a skincare expert. A weekly or bi-weekly exfoliating treatment or mask will help you to get further faster with your consistent routine, especially if your goal is brighter, less congested skin (or more even skin). But skin can often be over-exfoliated, and leaning on exfoliation for short-term results does not lend itself to long-term skin health.

Exfoliant recommendations:

* The REN Glycolactic Radiance Renewal Mask is packed with naturally derived glycolic and lactic acids (AHAs) and enzymes to motivate those dead skin cells to slough off. I'm a big fan of this one!

* For a heavy-hitter, the IMAGE Ageless Total Resurfacing Masque is chock-full of glycolic acid – often considered the most powerful exfoliating acid because of its small molecular sizing, which allows it to get deeper into the skin. For this same reason, glycolic acid can be more likely to exfoliate your skin *too* much, so go easy, listen to expert guidance and avoid if you have sensitive skin.

* Skingredients Sally Cleanser is a humdinger of a cleanser-exfoliator, packed with enough salicylic acid to encourage highly effective exfoliation while dissolving debris within the pore due to its oil-solubility. You only need to use this three times a week – about every third day. That's enough for it to do its job extremely well. A little of Sally goes a very long way.

* Malin + Goetz Brightening Enzyme Mask provides mild exfoliation for sensitive skins with enzymes and botanical AHAs. Enzymes exfoliate by gobbling up dead skin cells so it is difficult to over-exfoliate using enzymes, but it's still something to be wary of. This is best for those with sensitive skin, including those with rosacea.

* The Environ Focus Care Clarity+ Sebu-Clear Masque is ideal for those tackling congestion as it contains lactic acid for hydration and exfoliation plus salicylic acid and tea tree oil.

The Eighth Nerdie Principle

Good Skin Health is Habit-Forming

That one tiny word – habit – contains the success of all your skincare efforts. Good skincare is all about forming good, healthy habits when it comes to eating, cleansing and product application. I've read a theory that 21 repetitions is habit-forming. So by this logic, three weeks of consistent skincare should have you on your way to forming a reliable habit. And you can start slowly, making changes one by one, committing to each, monitoring the outcomes and using the results to cement your decision to keep going. You'll get to that lovely place where you do it almost without thinking – in fact, you'll feel all wrong if you *don't* do it. When it comes to good skin health, you want it to be the habit of a lifetime. And I'm going to do my bit by explaining exactly how it works and giving you the very rational and sound reasons why you should do it. You'll have no excuses then – you've been forewarned!

The daily skincare optionals

Spritzing

I adore spritzing my face throughout the day as it delivers the multiple benefits of hydrating and refreshing makeup, and sometimes they're antibacterial too. I may look like a diva doing it, but honestly, it's purely a functional thing! I spritz after cleansing, before applying serum to aid slip and penetration. And I often also spritz my body as opposed to moisturising with cream or body butter.

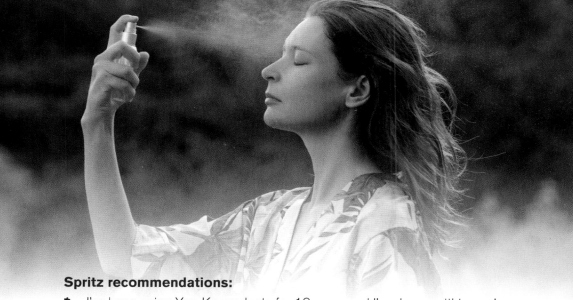

Spritz recommendations:

* I've been using Yon-Ka products for 12 years and I'm always within arm's length of a bottle of their Lotion Yon-Ka, either the PNG (normal or oily skin) or the PS (dry skin) format of the lotion.
* Avène Thermal Water Spray is fragrance-free, pure hydration.
* Murad Prebiotic 3-in-1 MultiMist has soothing prebiotics and tonnes of hydrators.
* Ella & Jo 3 in 1 Hyaluronic Skin Mist contains hyaluronic acid and soothers.
* Jane Iredale Pommisst has pomegranate extract, seaweed extract and white tea extract for antioxidant protection and mineral makeup refreshing.
* Caudalie Grape Water contains 100 per cent organic grape water, which is soothing and hydrating, and helps to reduce skin sensitivity.

Skincare supplements

In an ideal world, you would get all the nutrients you need to thrive from your diet. However, we have busy lives and can't guarantee that we'll manage to consume all the nutrients we need every day. This is where supplements can step in to help you maintain optimum nutrient levels.

I take skincare supplements daily because topical products can't physically penetrate the dermis, the deep living layer where skin forms. Skincare supplements feed the skin from within. Think of it as adding mulch to a rose bush – yes, the plant already has water, air and sun, but that little additional extra can make a big difference to how it thrives and blooms. I find supplements improve my mood, focus and attention.

Because I'm often asked, below I present to you the kinds of supplements I personally take daily:

Supplement type	Brand
Probiotic In my opinion, *everyone* should be taking probiotic supplements and yes, that includes you. There are studies that would agree with me and studies that would disagree, but I'm basing my opinion on my personal experience and the results I've witnessed first-hand with clients. However, I've been advised by many a nutritionist that the drinkable yoghurt-based ones are full of sugar as well as good bacteria. What you're looking for is a probiotic supplement where the probiotic can get to where it needs to be without being damaged by your stomach acid, and multiple bacteria strains can be key to look for too.	I take Symprove, a liquid dairy-free probiotic, because of the delivery system – it's water-based rather than freeze-dried so the live bacteria can get to the stomach without triggering digestion. Good digestive health is key to skin health as it means better absorption of nutrients, while helping with inflammation, gut health and serotonin levels. Other options are: ZENii Probiome Max are fantastic as they contain eight different bacterial strains for a full spectrum microbiome support. ANP Probiotics are great too. In their powder format, they can be sprinkled onto food.
Vitamin A Vitamin A is integral to your general skin health and it can be difficult to reach the optimum amount from diet alone – unless you are willing to chow down on eel or liver.	ANP Skin Vit A helps keep my skin clear. I also like Solgar Dry Vitamin A supplements.

Supplement type	Brand
Vitamin C Our bodies don't make vitamin C so it's super-important to ensure you are getting enough because it strengthens blood vessels (no more broken capillaries), prevents pigmentation and promotes collagen production. Fun fact: the only other creatures that don't make it themselves are guinea pigs.	Altrient C – this supplement has a scientifically proven liposomal delivery method (which means it's easier for the body to absorb and is carried to the cells directly without being damaged by the digestive system).
Omegas Essential fatty acids are key for the health of skin cell membranes and are believed to help with irritation and the skin's barrier.	Solgar Triple Strength Omegas – there's a notable difference in skin hydration and glow when I miss some.
Magnesium Research shows that it improves sleep, and sleep is vital for skin health as at night our skin heals, restores itself, becomes nourished, hydrates and exfoliates … everything we want it to do.	Biocare magnesium – for help with restful sleep when I need it.

If you feel you could benefit from targeted nutrient care, I recommend that you research it first and seek the advice of your GP, particularly if you are on any medication. Note that some supplements work well with others while some can block others from absorbing, so it's important to check this before taking anything. It's important to add too that you could potentially take an endless amount of supplements but this would be very expensive, take up a lot of time and won't necessarily have the impact you want. In the end, the choice will depend on your skin concerns and circumstances. As with every part of our skincare approach, keeping it consistent and relevant to your concerns is the goal.

Some people believe that supplements are unnecessary, but I disagree. I'm not in the habit of doing anything that isn't targeted and beneficial when it comes to spending money and time on my skin. I see the difference, as do our Nerd Network members. The brands I work with are fact-driven, with scientific data behind them, and we have also spoken to thousands of people online over the years who report good results.

Supplements are an investment, complementing your healthy diet. Ideally, we would get all the nutrition we need from our diet, but the key skin nutrients – vitamin A, omegas and vitamin C – can be hard to get in the right amounts through food. We may hit the recommended daily allowance, which basically aims to stop us from getting ill, but we struggle to get the optimal daily amount.

And poor gut bacteria, alcohol, caffeine and smoking (or vaping … any form of tobacco product) can get in the way of nutrient absorption. Supplements ensure that you have the maximum amount of nutrients to keep feeding your skin (the healthier you are, the more impact they'll have) and good-quality supplements are *specifically designed* to get to where they need to go without being damaged or depleted.

Skincare supplement recommendations:

Skin problem	Supplement recommendation
Smoking	It's believed that smoking can deplete vitamin C. Ideally, for skin health and general health, quitting smoking is the best option. If this is something you're still working towards, you may need to up your dietary intake of vitamin C or opt for a supplement.
Redness	Probiotics, vitamin C for capillary health and omegas to help with inflammation.

Skin problem	Supplement recommendation
Acne	Probiotics, vitamin A, DIM, zinc and omegas for inflammation (zinc is also known to aid with healing ability) and skin hydration. **Ensure that you are not getting more than the upper limit of vitamin A between your diet and supplements as this can cause adverse effects. Those taking Roaccutane (Accutane) should not take vitamin A supplements, as RoAccutane is a form of vitamin A. Additionally, you should not take vitamin A supplements while pregnant – follow the advice of your GP or healthcare provider.
Dryness	Omegas are recommended if your skin is dry, dehydrated or if you have eczema, rosacea or other conditions where your skin's barrier has become compromised. The supplement should be good quality, i.e. Epax certified. Solgar and Hush & Hush have vegan options so those who don't consume animal products can get those fats in.
Ageing	Vitamin C, antioxidant supplement such as Solgar Curcumin or ANP Skin Antioxidant to protect from the inside, anti-ageing supplements like ANP Skin Youth Biome (probiotics plus vitamin C) or ANP Skin Collagen Support which combines vitamins A, C and D.

Your busy life skincare routines

So many clients have said to me, 'I don't like my skin, but I don't have time to do anything about it.' Well, the truth is, yes, you do. If you have the time to watch Netflix, you have time for your skin, trust me. Commit to yourself by dedicating a short (achievable) period of time to skincare every evening. And we're going to start with a one-minute routine, which is time you can definitely spare for the good of your skin. (I haven't included time to put on makeup here, but that's your call.)

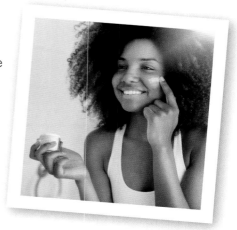

First, let's take a moment to look at how you apply the products. I'll repeat my key mantra here: apply from the nipples up. Start massaging in the product just above the nipples, then work up over the neck, onto the face, through the eyebrows and into the hairline, out to the ears, behind the ears. Don't forget the whole under-chin area. Cleansing from the nipples up is essential, especially for those blessed with larger busts and pronounced cleavage. Work that décolletage!

The one-minute A.M. routine (our three steps)

* Cleanse for 30 seconds with Cleanse Off Mitt, mild (passive) cleanser and water.
* Use a serum (a vitamin A would be the core recommendation but if pregnant and your preferred serum is not suitable for use, you can use a hydrating antioxidant product).
* Apply SPF – make sure it has a moisturising effect.
* Done!
* BUT – if your skin only got a very cursory cleanse last night for whatever reason, what can you do in the morning? I recommend a thorough cleanse – Skingredients PreProbiotic Cleanse would work well, for example, to hydrate the skin and perform a slight exfoliation to get the skin back on track.

The aim here is very simple: to clean and protect. This routine may not bring about colossal skin changes – unless you opt to use a vitamin A serum – but it will get you into a good skincare habit, and then you can build on that.

The one-minute P.M. routine

Are rules made to be broken? When it comes to skin – no! But I understand that some nights you might be just too exhausted for a lengthy routine. (The less said about the reasons why this might be, the better!) If this is how you're feeling, you still can't skip the routine, so I recommend you repeat the one-minute A.M. routine and fall into bed. And you get to skip a step, because you don't need SPF at night. You can handle that!

The two-minute A.M. routine

* Pre-cleanse with COM.
* Cleanse for 60 seconds with your mild (passive) cleanser and COM.
* Apply serum. You might wish to use two serums and mix them together. If you do, mix a small amount of both on the palm of your hand and apply. Think of it as a base ingredient and a skin-specific ingredient, e.g. if you need more hydration, then add a hydrating serum to your all-rounder serum. A common combination would be a vitamin A serum and a brightening serum.
* Apply SPF.

The two-minute P.M. routine

* The exact same as your two-minute A.M., but swap your cleanser out for an active cleanser (as per recommendation – i.e. once every three days).
* Apply your serums.
* No SPF needed.

This is a standard core routine, and if you're using the right ingredients and products, you're going to see results. Most people don't need much more than this – super minimal, minimal buy-in, minimal shelf space required and still decent results … so long as you stick to it daily. Consistency is key!

The five-minute A.M. routine

* Pre-cleanse
* Cleanse for 60 seconds – same as the two-minute routine.
* Apply your serums as in the two-minute A.M. routine but spend more time doing it and try to incorporate some deep exhales, like in the Wim Hof Method as noted by Níall Ó Murchú earlier (page 52). It's best to use whichever product has more slip to incorporate some facial massage movements for two minutes for lymphatic drainage.
* Apply your SPF!

The five-minute P.M. routine

* Pre-cleanse with your COM and mild cleanser.
* Cleanse with your exfoliating cleanser for 60 seconds.
* Apply your serums, same as the A.M. routine, with the same breathing techniques.
* Incorporate some facial massage movements (see page 241 of *The Skin Nerd* or our Instagram page for tips) using a facial oil, such as the Codex Beauty Bia Facial Oil.
* Finish with a night cream, if you need one.

The ten-minute in-shower routine

Why just stand in the shower when you can use this time for an effective and time-busting skincare routine? I mean, you're in there in the nip anyway, so why not put all that bare skin to good use?

* First off, a good dry body brushing before you turn the shower on. Brush towards your heart with light motions to get the lymphatic system pumping.
* Pre-cleanse with your COM or a pre-cleanse balm.
* If you fancy doing a face mask, apply an acid-based exfoliating mask.
* Cleanse – switch off the shower for a moment (to save water) and apply cleansers from the nipples up. If you are doing this step in the shower

and you have a few minutes to spare, it would be a good idea to add in some very basic destressing massage movements. (See our IGTVs on Instagram for tips on how to do this.) So, massage the eye area outwards using your ring finger, pressing on the bone, which helps with depuffing. Then press across your eyebrows using your thumb and middle finger. If you suffer with sinus issues, press along them, including the pocket beside the nose, using your forefinger flat onto the face and tap in a pulsing rhythm. Then turn the shower back on – water warm, not hot – and cleanse away the mask.

* Body cleanse – it's easy to remember to do the legs, torso and arms, but often the back gets forgotten and it can be prone to spots. Apply treatment cleanser to your back, including on your bum and top of thighs as these areas are prone to sweating. If you're thinking a shower companion/servant is going to be one of my essential ingredients for this, relax! I have another solution. You can attach a COM to something like a spatula to reach all those tricky places. This homemade solution is better than shower scrubbers or pompoms for the simple reason that people often don't clean those regularly, making them breeding grounds for bacteria, whereas it's easy to remove the COM and clean it. Finally, don't forget to

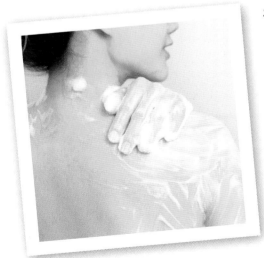

wash the bottom of your feet as well. Sit down to do this, if necessary – and safety first, don't slip getting back up. (Note: don't apply acid products and shave that skin area on the same day.)

* Turn off the water and congratulate yourself for efficient use of your shower time.

* If you love a body moisturiser, go for it – but remember to apply it to wet skin. Personally, I prefer to spritz after showering because it's not sticky. I find a good balanced diet

full of essential fatty acids means a body moisturiser is not as necessary but I do keep a body moisturiser handy for those typical elephant knees and elbows that can crop up.

The Saturday indulgence 'me-time' routine

This is particularly good to do after a long, hard week, when skin needs a little extra help anyway. It's also nice to do as a bedtime routine, to calm you down and prepare you for a good night's sleep, which is of course a skin treatment all by itself.

* Lock the bathroom door, take a deep breath. Yep, you're alone in a quiet space. Enjoy!
* If you fancy a shower, hop in. (One quick bummer of a note: hot showers aren't recommended because they can remove the skin's protective oils, leading to red, itchy, flaky, irritated skin. But if you only do it once in a while, I can avert my nerdie eye.) Then wrap yourself in a soft towel and enjoy giving your skin some TLC.
* Pre-cleanse your face with a COM and warm water to prep your skin.
* Use a pre-cleanse balm, such as the Dermalogica Precleanse Balm. This will remove oils and any debris from the skin so everything that follows will be able to penetrate the skin easily. Remove this balm thoroughly, as oils can prevent other ingredients from soaking in.
* Cleanse with a treatment cleanser, such as one with glycolic acid, salicylic acid or vitamin C, whatever works best for your skin.
* Exfoliate – your second helping of exfoliation can be a mask such as the Drunk Elephant TLC Sukari Babyfacial or an exfoliating powder like the IMAGE Iluma Intense Brightening Exfoliating Powder or Dermalogica Daily Microfoliant.
* Apply serum(s) – you may be a monogamous serum user, or you may like to do it with a couple at a time. No judgement here (in fact, this is encouraged!). If using two serums (for general and specific targeting),

mix them in the palm of your hand after removing your exfoliant or mask. Make sure to massage in gently.

* Moisturise – an optional step if you have a moisturiser that you love and that works for your skin. Before using around the eyes, check the label to make sure it's suitable for this.
* Massage with a light facial oil, such as the Bia Facial Oil from Codex Beauty. Oil will give some necessary slip while you massage, allowing your fingers to glide rather than drag. If it's daytime, remove the oil afterwards with a quick cleanse – you can also pat off excess oil with a clean piece of tissue. If you're heading straight to bed, leave the oil on to absorb into the skin. Or, if you prefer, you can use a leave-on sheet mask overnight.
* As for the rest of your body, apply a good body moisturiser or oil rich in vitamins and/or ceramides while the skin is still damp.

And if you're doing this pre-bed rather than on Saturday morning, follow these instructions:

* PJs on.
* Dim the lights.
* Relax! You've done a whole lot of good for your skin, it feels fresh, gorgeous and you deserve a good night's sleep.

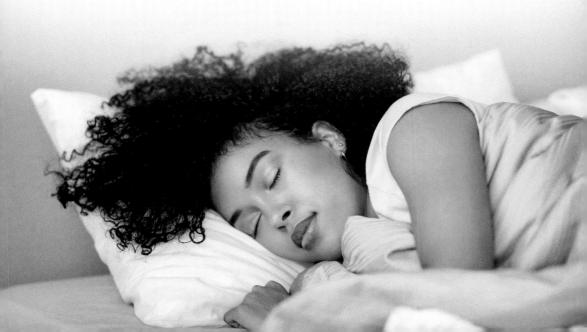

My treatment guide

If treatments aren't something you've explored before, here's a brief guide to the most popular types and my own take on them.

Treatment	Description	Benefits
LED	Light-emitting diode (LED) therapy works to target skin concerns like congestion, ageing and inflammation with different-coloured light pulsed into the skin.	Depending on the colour of the light, it can kill bacteria, promote skin healing, soothe the skin and promote regeneration of the skin.
Peels	Chemical peels work to rapidly increase skin cell turnover for fresh skin; depending on the acids and ingredients used within them, they may have different results. All peels are not the same, advanced qualifications will allow different depths of peels, different brands will offer ingredients with different purposes. A peel also does not always mean the skin should peel!	A salicylic acid peel will reduce oil production, dissolve debris within the pores, target active acne and help to prevent it; an AHA peel will help to reduce the appearance of ageing, pigment and texture. The acids vary depending on skin concern, activity, whether they are buffered, or non-buffered (meaning whether the pH is adjusted for efficacy or not); brand to brand, it all differs and no two peels are the same.
Microneedling (Also known as dermarolling or collagen stimulation therapy)	Fine needles prick the skin, triggering what is known as the healing cascade, stimulating production of collagen, elastin and growth factors.	Newer skin, improved texture, improvement in scarring (pigment or textural), anti-ageing.

Doesn't work for …	Personally speaking …
It's safe for all	I adore LED and believe it to be a fantastic modality, especially for those who cannot take much stimulation on the skin – e.g. those with rosacea.
Those with sensitive skin	I rate light-level, non-aggressive peels when they are performed often – i.e. a lower percentage regularly rather than a higher percentage done as a once off. Please note that, confusingly enough, peels don't always cause the skin to visibly shed. Enzymatic peels in particular will gently slough off the dead skin cells due to turn over at that period.
Those with active acne, those with rosacea, eczema or other medical skin conditions associated with inflammation.	I am a huge advocate for microneedling, having practised it and having had it carried out frequently – it brings about noticeable results quickly, but it's key that skin is healthy first as this will offer better results.

Treatment	Description	Benefits
Meso needling	Fine, shorter needles than microneedling, used to enhance absorption of ingredients such as hyaluronic acid which is applied during the treatment	Depending on the product applied during meso needling – it could be better hydration, glowier, fresher skin, improved circulation – in my opinion, it's great for short-term results. Meso needling is key for those looking for more instant results, i.e. in the lead-up to a big event such as a wedding.
Microdermabrasion	Available in either crystal format or diamond-tipped, indeed it's often used as the first step in a treatment as opposed to a stand-alone treatment.	It tends to buff off the top layer – i.e. the stratum corneum – which mechanically allows for the skin to feel smooth, fresh and even in appearance and texture immediately.

Doesn't work for ...	Personally speaking ...
Those with active acne, those with rosacea, eczema or other medical skin conditions associated with inflammation.	Meso needling is a great technique for assisting in ingredient penetration when a serum or ampoule is applied. Many experts believe repetitive meso needling will have a similar impact to microneedling over a longer period of time.
Those with active acne, sensitive skin, eczema, other medical conditions associated with inflammation, those with a compromised barrier, broken capillaries, fragile skin or crêpey skin.	It is superficial and at times can be, in my opinion, quite abrasive on the skin. I tend to endorse treatments such as mild peels in lieu of this treatment as they will also give the immediate satisfactory sensation while potentially triggering the collagen and elastin at a cellular level, not just ones we can touch and feel. I think it can be beneficial as part of treatments such as HydraFacial or when used alongside IPL or peels, but I don't rate it highly as a stand-alone treatment.

The Ninth Nerdie Principle

Trends Do Not Usually Justify the Means

Think about looking back at old pics, times when you thought you looked so cool. The brows! (We'll say nothing!) Remember how much money you spent on those low-rise jeans? Cringe-worthy memories, no? They all have something in common – you followed a trend. It wasn't really for you, but you threw caution to the wind and told yourself it was made for you … but you were wrong. Trends are not always your friend – especially when it comes to skincare. Every year, a new 'it product' becomes all the rage and the next thing you know, it's 'over' and the next big thing is waiting in the wings. At their worst, trends can compromise your skin health. But on the positive side, trends can also be exciting new technologies or products that become mainstays because of how effective they are. I'm a devoted believer in figuring out what works for your skin and sticking to it, regardless of what's hot or not right now. The end goal is healthy skin – the means are the best practices and formulations to help you achieve that. And those means shouldn't change just because a celebrity says you should be massaging bird excrement into your face. Go with what you know, go with how your skin feels, then you can't go wrong.

Chapter 10

The Skin Professional Jigsaw Puzzle

You can now recite, by heart, the most important nerdie philosophy: good skincare must involve a three-pronged 360° approach: inside (mindset and diet), outside (including traditional skincare with active and passive steps) and on top (SPF protection and makeup, if using). We also need to keep in mind that the skin is an organ (did I mention this?) that encompasses the lymphatic system, muscle and skin layers. Even though these components are interlinked, they each require their own targeted help and nothing – no wonder drug, no promises with exclamation marks, no one-stop-shop elixir – can work on all of them successfully.

Thankfully, the skinformation available today is highly detailed, giving a really broad view of what our skin is, how it works and what it needs from us to do its job well. (And we're talking head-to-toe skin here, none of this 'face first' business.) This suits me perfectly because I've been shouting about holistic skincare for a long time. I live by it myself, which means I am my own walking experiment and laboratory and, even though there are good skin days and not so good days, the results are inarguable.

But adopting such a broad approach can be daunting for many of us. Good skincare habits seem to involve so many moving parts that need to be balanced consistently, even after the initial habit has been established. And the vast array of skincare advice and skin professionals out there can be mighty puzzling. It might even stop you from seeking out help if you feel you're facing some kind of skincare labyrinth that's impossible to make your way round – or out of! But I am here to help. This chapter is all about providing you with the information you need to navigate this confusion easily and get to where you'll find the best solution for your skin.

So, speaking of puzzles, here's one I prepared earlier: a helpful jigsaw puzzle of experts, all with different areas of expertise when it comes to skin health.

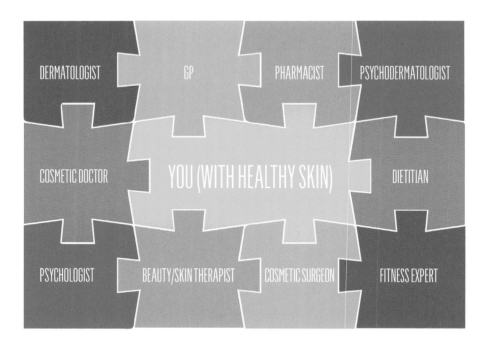

When it comes to experts, as with all the information I'm sharing in this book, there's no point simply listing who they are – you need to know how these disciplines can work together to address *your* skindividual needs. If you're trying to target skin concerns from all angles but feeling unsure or daunted about where to start, it's helpful to know that there is a network of professionals, medical and aesthetic, who can work together to provide you with a tailor-made 360° plan. And it's important to remember that there are some conditions, such as severe acne, that cannot be treated by topical skincare alone. Choosing to go it alone can compromise your skin health, and your mental health as well in the long run. There's no need to feel alone and at the mercy of your skin condition – there are so many people out there who can help you.

But what does your skin need? It all depends on where you're starting from and where you want to end up. It might be a dash of dietary advice, a healthy portion of guidance from skin experts, a few trips to a dermatologist or a visit to check in with your GP. Or you might require complementary input from a number of different experts, maybe even some not detailed here, such as an endocrinologist for hormonal problems. Good experts are respectful of each other's roles and will work together towards one common goal: helping you to achieve improved confidence and health.

The first step is figuring out who can best help you.

Do I Need to Seek Expert Help and Which Expert Do I Consult?

The million-dollar question. Generally, there are two types of people when it comes to skin issues. There are those who register a skin concern and try to sort it as soon as possible. Then there are those who ignore it, praying it will disappear of its own accord, whispering incantations to the gods of clear skin … until it worsens. Unsurprisingly, the ones who hop to it are always better off because the sooner you can acknowledge that you need some help, the sooner you can start working on the (sometimes long) process of sorting out the problem. My advice is to seek help as soon as you notice a problem that you don't feel you can manage on your own, or that you feel is out of the ordinary for you. The issue is not going to improve if you do nothing. Or there might not be a concern at all – some people would just like some general guidance about good skin health. Either way, you are in control. Help the experts to help you. It's also very important to make sure that you find the correct expert for your concern and that you have a natural alignment with them, that you feel safe and have faith in their care.

So, who you gonna call? These skin-issue busters:

You should seek the help of a skin therapist if:

* you are lost and confused about what to purchase, the sector is confusing to you and you're not sure which route to take
* you want additional skin health advice alongside the advice of a GP, dermatologist or dietitian. FYI, a skin therapist is a professional with a qualification in beauty therapy who has continued to specialise in skin – they may be a facialist, skincare consultant or both (whereas a dermatologist has a medical qualification). Skin therapy is often neglected in this jigsaw puzzle, but for aesthetic results and for ongoing skin health, skin therapists can be essential guides and can bring about great results. It's well worth becoming acquainted with their perspective and treatments.
* you want to deal with puffiness
* your skin is too dry
* you want to improve your skin texture
* you suffer from excessive oiliness, blackheads and small whiteheads
* you want to maintain skin health and prevent the signs of accelerated ageing
* you see mild redness that you don't believe to be a symptom of rosacea
* you have skin pigmentation that isn't related to hormones (melasma and chloasma due to hormonal fluctuations or during pregnancy or won't be affected by typical skincare routines for pigmentation).

You should seek the help of a GP if:

* what you're experiencing is medical as opposed to a visual or aesthetic concern
* your acne or congestion is persistent, inflamed and sore
* your acne is greatly affecting your mental health
* you suspect you could be suffering from eczema
* you suspect you could be suffering from psoriasis
* you suspect you could be suffering from rosacea
* you are unsure what your skin concern is
* you have a mole or patch of skin that has suddenly changed
* you have been recommended to speak to your GP by a skin therapist or dietitian.

You should speak to a dietitian if:

* your skin concern seems to be linked with dietary factors (i.e. you break out only when you eat dairy, or your rosacea is triggered by spicy food)
* in the past you have tried all other means, such as topical skincare, antibiotics and other treatments
* you want to improve your skin through your diet and are confident about your topical skin routine
* you have been recommended to speak to a dietitian by your GP or by a skin therapist.

You should speak to a dermatologist if:

* you have been advised to do this by your GP, a skin therapist, or a dietitian – although note that only GPs can make a referral
* your skin concern is persistent, even after following GP treatment and/or treatment from a skin therapist or dietitian.

You should speak to a mental health expert if:

* you are experiencing anxiety or stress of any kind that you feel might be contributing to your poor physical health
* your feelings about your skin are affecting your mood, confidence or self-esteem.

You should speak to a fitness expert/personal trainer if:

* you want to enhance skin health through exercise – physical exercise is key for body and mental health and so in turn for skin health
* you are nervous about joining a gym and your ability to undertake exercise
* you are overweight and wish to lose weight – if this is the case for you, it's a good idea to talk to your GP first and discuss the options regarding healthy and safe weight loss.

Over to the Experts!

You'll know by now that I hugely respect the opinions of experts and value their input. That's why I've invited a number of different experts to take over this chapter and give you the benefit of their expertise. I'm not an expert in each of these disciplines, so I'll step back (which is very hard for me to do, I admit!) and let them impart their wisdom to you.

You'll now hear from:

1. a psychodermatologist

2. a psychologist

3. a dietitian

4. a fitness expert

5. a skin therapist

THE SKIN NERD PHILOSOPHY

6 an LED machine expert

7 an industry expert

8 CEO of the British Beauty Council

9 a pharmacist

10 a GP

11 a cosmetic doctor

12 a cosmetic surgeon

13 a dermatologist

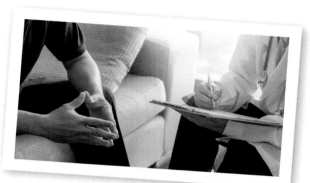

The psychodermatologist

We've already touched upon psychodermatology in Chapter 3, where I described the links between brain, gut and skin and their effect on skin health. Psychodermatologist Dr Alia Ahmed cares deeply about the psychosocial effects of skin conditions, which can often be neglected, because skin concerns are sometimes believed to be related solely to aesthetics or vanity. Highly educated, extremely dedicated, professional and, most of all, hooman and approachable, Dr Ahmed is holistic in her approach to medicine, which I find so progressive and appealing. Here she gives us an expert's insight into this intriguing branch of skin thought.

How may our mental health contribute to common skin concerns or conditions?

There is increasing evidence to suggest that patients with dermatological disease have higher levels of psychological and psychiatric issues than those with other chronic diseases. My patients often tell me that their skin is impacting the way they feel and vice versa. In fact, 85% of dermatology patients feel that psychosocial factors are a major component of their illness, and 17% need psychological support to cope with their condition. Thirty per cent of people with skin disease have high levels of psychological distress. Worryingly, there is increasing evidence that people with a skin condition are engaging in suicidal behaviours, rather than being able to live with their diagnosis. There is evidence to show that addressing psychological factors can improve outcomes for people with skin conditions.

A large proportion of the patients I see include those with chronic skin disease (e.g. acne, rosacea, vitiligo) that has a psychological impact (e.g. low self-esteem/body confidence, social anxiety and depression), and those with conditions that are impacted by stress (e.g. eczema, psoriasis, urticaria). In addition, I see patients whose skin problems are rooted in psychiatric or psychological distress (e.g. chronic itch, hair pulling, skin picking, nail biting and body dysmorphia).

How does stress affect our skin? What are the knock-on effects on our skin's vital processes?

Stress and skin are closely linked; I often say to my patients 'stress causes skin disease and skin disease causes stress'. The well-established link between mind and skin can be explained at a biochemical level via the Hypothalamic-Pituitary-Adrenal (HPA) axis. Stress activates this neuroendocrine system which causes activation and dysregulation of cellular processes that cause or drive skin disease (especially inflammatory, autoimmune or allergic skin conditions). Feelings of emotional distress lead to the release of a stress hormone (cortisol), which is known to affect the immune system (making the skin less able to defend itself), drive allergic responses, delay healing and disrupt the skin's natural barrier (leading to loss of water and natural moisturising factors). The effects seen on the skin can vary, including feeling red, dry and itchy, as well as the formation of lines, wrinkles, pigmentation, signs of premature ageing and dull skin. The role of stress is well known to cause or drive skin conditions like eczema, psoriasis, alopecia, urticaria, acne breakouts and skin tumours. Short-term stress (e.g. feeling anxious before a presentation/exam) can cause temporary problems like flushing, itching and sweating. Long-term (or chronic) stress, however, results in the body entering a permanent 'stress-response' state, which can aggravate existing skin problems through a poor natural immune response and ongoing inflammation. For example, high levels of stress are associated with a higher severity of skin disease in people with psoriasis and eczema.

How do we see body dysmorphia manifest when it comes to skin concerns, appearance and conditions, and what can be done?

Body dysmorphic disorder (BDD) is a condition where the individual has a disproportionate concern or preoccupation with a real or imagined defect related to their physical appearance. This is a very real and debilitating concern, and it can lead to several symptoms including low mood, social anxiety and withdrawal from people and relationships. People with BDD will check their appearance in mirrors multiple times a day, repeatedly compare themselves with others, seek reassurance, avoid social interactions, spend excessive time concealing 'flaws', and they can feel ugly or deformed. The impact of these appearance-related concerns causes significant psychological distress and functional impairment (e.g. avoiding social situations, occupational difficulties, relationship problems). BDD is associated with disorders like anxiety and major depression, as well as obsessive and suicidal behaviours and substance misuse. A number of these patients will present to aesthetic or skincare practitioners and may be missing out on important medical management of their skin concern.

An example of a patient in this category is someone who has mild acne but is so upset by it they have stopped socialising with their friends, spend hours in front of the mirror examining their skin, feel low and depressed about the way they look, in extreme cases leading to suicidal thoughts. My job in this scenario is to treat the acne appropriately but also explore why it is such a problem for the individual concerned. It is important to spend time establishing a relationship with the patient and then to be able to highlight the negative impact of their appearance-related concerns on their quality of life. Combination treatment with antidepressants and cognitive behavioural therapy has shown to have good treatment outcomes for people with BDD.

The psychologist

Senior psychologist and chartered psychologist of the Psychological Society of Ireland Dr Clíodhna O'Donovan gives her expert view on the often-overlooked mind–skin aspect of skincare. Dr O'Donovan is particularly interested in skin (and skincare) in her personal life, and is a regular consultant for information on self-esteem, self-confidence and mental health for *Stellar* magazine.

Can you talk us through the mind–skin link?

For me, thinking about self-esteem with regard to skin has personal salience. It's our largest organ, and we wear it all the time so how it looks can impact on how comfortable we feel in ourselves. A bad skin day may go hand-in-hand with thoughts like, 'I look awful today. I hope I don't bump into anyone.' This is intensified even more for those with underlying self-esteem issues and for whom their appearance is inextricably linked to their sense of self-worth. In this age of filters, many of us crave perfection and 'the Photoshop effect', which of course is not how our skin actually looks. However, someone might begin to believe 'I'm only a person of value if my skin looks perfect', that the skin must look like it has been mildly filtered at all times, thereby setting unrealistic goals about one's appearance, not to mention the negative consequences for self-esteem.

No one, psychologists included, is immune to these thoughts or feelings. Furthermore, having a negative relationship with your skin is not just reserved for acne-prone adolescents – many people at every stage in life (and of any gender) can experience this, due to fine lines, rosacea or other skin problems. This can manifest in a number of ways – you might look down because of a blemish on your chin, or you feel like your fine lines are more pronounced and you don't want to make eye contact. While we all have days where we feel less comfortable with our appearance, if it becomes a pattern whereby your view of your skin and your appearance in general are negatively impacting on your self-esteem, this is where you may benefit from attending a suitably qualified psychologist or therapist to explore these issues further, in a bid to improve your relationship with yourself and develop a greater sense of self-compassion.

You might want your skin to be perfect all the time, I certainly know I do, and that's fine, but you shouldn't feel any less worthy or less loveable today because you're having a bad skin day, compared to last week or yesterday when your skin looked good. You're human, your hormones fluctuate, you may have eaten something that didn't agree with you and that's all okay.

Therapy can often be about supporting a person to hold together two seemingly opposing concepts: in this context it may be how to help you feel better about the skin that you currently have, while also knowing it's okay to want to improve your skin, as long as you have a compassionate acceptance of yourself as you are and don't feel any lesser if your skin isn't in tip-top condition. This fundamental message needs to be managed sensitively, delivered in the context of a supportive, therapeutic relationship. Furthermore, as a therapist, understanding a person's personal struggles, whatever they may be, and wanting those things to improve for them is a perfect example of empathy. It's like saying, 'I understand that your skin is a big concern for you and you really want it to get better and I really want that for you too and also I am accepting of you just as you are, as a person of inherent value and worth, regardless of how your skin appears.'

This process is like holding together all the parts of the skin jigsaw and may involve directing a client to allied professionals who have the necessary skills to support the client on their skin journey, be that their GP who may suggest a referral to a dermatologist, dietitian or other skin specialist. Aside from the aesthetic side, problematic skin may be indicative of other underlying health concerns for which I do not have the training nor qualifications to investigate nor treat but by directing my clients to discuss their concerns with their GP or other health professional so these concerns can be investigated fully.

The dietitian

I asked expert dietitian Orla Walsh to advise us on the diet aspect of the inside-out approach to skin health. My intrigue is always piqued at internal skin health and fuelling the organ with food.

When it comes to improving your skin, a holistic approach is necessary. When you work with a team of lots of different healthcare professionals, each coming from a different angle and with a different point of view, more can be achieved. Generally, treatment tends to be more thorough. For example, if someone comes in for an appointment with me and I notice something about their skin that requires more investigation, I'd refer back to their GP. A dietitian would be able to recognise a skin problem associated with, to give an example, undiagnosed coeliac disease, and they would suggest that person go back to their GP, request a blood test and investigate whether your assumption is correct. If needed then, the GP will refer on to another member of a team, like a gastroenterologist.

Another example would be if someone came in and showed signs that they may have polycystic ovary syndrome. You may again refer back to their GP, who'd test their hormones. If their skin concerns are hormone related and the GP gives a diagnosis of PCOS, then they might be referred on to a gynaecologist and/or an endocrinologist.

In the inverse, many healthcare professionals would refer on to a dietitian. If someone had a skin issue that was due to an allergy, they may refer to a dietitian so that proper exclusion of the allergen can take place and that no nutritional gaps are formed. They also might refer on to a dietitian if they feel that dietetic input may help. Some nutrients are very important in the management of eczema, or an anti-inflammatory diet might help with psoriasis.

10% of women are reported to have PCOS, and PCOS can impact someone's skin and increase the risk of acne. Dietary management in PCOS is super important, both to manage the PCOS symptoms as well as the condition. If you manage your PCOS through diet, this can have significant improvements on your skin. Some professionals might refer to a dietitian to help manage a diet when they know that diet can have a large impact on the management of the skin condition in question.

Diet is important in the management of acne. The likely approach that someone would take would be to put that person on a low glycaemic load diet, assess for triggers and see if certain food or food groups exacerbate this skin *condition as well as look at making sure the diet is nutritionally complete so that the skin is being fed from the inside out.*

The fitness expert

Next up, we have personal trainer Karl Henry to give us some words of encouragement. I've had the pleasure of speaking with Karl on his Real Health podcast after years of admiring his work, ethos and philosophy on *Operation Transformation*. His well-rounded approach, with nutritionally balanced food plans and classic, motivated hard work, has changed lives.

Okay so hands up, I am no skin expert. Exercise and helping people to get in the best shape possible is what I do. Each and every client I have had in my 20 years of personal training has seen one very common benefit from getting more exercise in: improved skin. As part of a regime that includes eating better, using the recommended skincare and professional advice, it's incredibly empowering to see what a big difference moving more can make to your skin.

You see, your skin is the largest organ the body has and organs need blood flow along with removal of waste products and exercise does exactly that. Increased blood flow through exercise brings more oxygen and nutrients to the skin cells and helps to remove waste products. Makes sense to think that this can benefit the skin, doesn't it?

People tend to focus on the cardiovascular benefits of physical activity, and those are important, but any movement that promotes healthy circulation also helps keep your skin healthy and glowing. Remember, that's any exercise: weights, Pilates, cardio, tai chi … Just the process of moving more will make a big difference to your skin.

Increasing that blood flow and removing waste is a direct benefit of movement, but don't forget the indirect benefits:

1. *Reduction in stress levels*
2. *Better sleep*
3. *Improved mood*

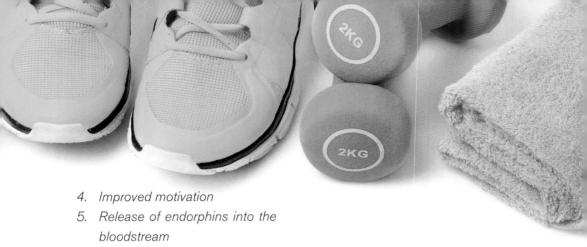

4. *Improved motivation*
5. *Release of endorphins into the bloodstream*
6. *Overall sense of wellbeing*

All of the above will improve your skin, and the beauty of it is that they are free benefits of movement that generally can be free too, so it's a win-win all round.

Okay, but what if you have dermatological conditions such as acne, rosacea, or psoriasis? Should you still exercise?

Firstly, I would say that getting professional skin advice is important here as each person is different, but also try these tips:

* *Do a deep skin clean before the workout so that you are exercising with a clean face.*
* *Aim to exercise in an area that is cool and well-ventilated.*
* *Avoid exercising at the hottest part of the day.*
* *Ensure you are keeping hydrated during the workout.*
* *Use soft fabrics to wipe away sweat.*
* *If you suffer from chafing, aim for clothes that are breathable, avoid cotton fabrics and use Vaseline or Bodyglide on the affected areas.*

Finally, remember that exercise makes you feel good. That sense of confidence, achievement and completing something gives you almost a glow. It's a tangible feeling that you know you did well. That alone will improve your skin, combined with all the other benefits above. Listen to skin and nutrition experts, get some movement in and you're rocking! Skin health is about combining lots of different parts of your life, getting advice where you need it, and then that jigsaw of advice and lifestyle fitting together to get your skin looking its very, very best.

The skin therapist

I have long known of skincare specialist Jeanne Brophy and held her professionalism, willingness and constant need to learn as the reason why she is truly the go-to facialist in Ireland.

What is the most effective treatment you can have in a clinic or salon?
There are so many amazing new technologies and treatments on the market, but in my opinion, there is no clear winner because each skin has different needs, and what will work beautifully for one may not for someone else. A multi-modality approach is key. Ideally, work with someone who will set a plan for your skin using a blend of treatments. In my experience, this is the best path to long-term skin health. There are so many treatments available, it is difficult to list one as the best for certain complaints, but the below will give an overview of some really effective treatments for each concern.

After a few weeks on a prescribed home care plan, I think it is always good to start with a few facials tailored to your skin. This will gently lift dead cells, infuse hydration and create a good base for any stronger treatments you may need. The basic cleanse, tone and mask facial is gone, and bespoke facials can contain anything from meso needling, microcurrent, gentle peels and light therapy. They will always have massage elements, which are so important to keep circulation and tone in your skin. Massage, both at home and in your professional treatments, is a must!

For congested skin, salicylic acid facials or peels are really effective. Salicylic helps to mop up excess dead skin and oils that accumulate in the pore causing congestion. Congestion is a natural part of having an oily skin, so for those who struggle, a home care vitamin A-based product is key to help manage this. This can range from mild to prescription, depending on your needs.

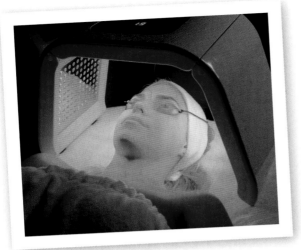

Many clients start focusing more on scars or enlarged pores on their skin when their oil has become more managed. Microneedling is a great next step here. It stimulates the skin to produce collagen, which helps rejuvenate it. This can help to reduce the appearance of open pores or marking, leading to a more even complexion. Whilst closing open pores is not an option, it does help to reduce the appearance and definitely helps overall skin health. It's a favourite of mine for many skins and gives really great results. Clinics offer this treatment in a roller or pen system, both of which are very effective.

For redness, step one is to get any sensitivity or reactiveness issues under control. This is often done through home care and facials. I love the Environ facials for this. The sonophoresis machine used by Environ helps to infuse ingredients into the skin whilst protecting the barrier, which is really important if you have a more reactive skin. LED light therapy is also excellent. It is a gentle but effective way of rejuvenating a sensitive skin and gives really nice results. Light can go where hands can't, so it's a great way of stimulating the deeper layers of the skin without irritating it. The machine is very relevant, though, so it's worth looking into how strong the machine used is before signing up to a course of treatments. Dermalux is my favourite. Professionally, the smaller units unfortunately just don't have enough energy to give adequate results. [See pages 192–193 for more information on LED treatments.]

If specific vessels or veins on your skin are the main concern, IPL [Intense Pulsed Light treatment] is the best way to target these. A course of treatments will often be needed for best results and ongoing top-up treatments will be needed to maintain the result.

When it comes to pigmentation and uneven skin tone, I think doing what we can to help keep an even complexion is a must as we get older. An even *complexion is always youthful and has a better light reflection so makes it easier to create the glow we all want as skin ages. Home care and facial treatments are perfect if you are at the prevention, mild or possibly moderate stage, but if things have moved on from there, or you want faster results, there are other options.*

Mild pigmentation: *combine home care, LED therapy, meso needling (a milder version of microneedling which can be used with specific serums to help lighten surface pigment), bespoke facials and lightening peels.*

Severe pigmentation: *there are a number of options that can be done. Home care routines from a dermatologist using tretinoin and hydroquinone can be very effective. These should only be used for a shorter period of time and should only ever be done in consultation with your dermatologist. The Mesoestetic Cosmelan Peel or Dermaceutic Mela Peel are also very effective options for more severe pigment.*

If your concern is skin laxity, I think massage is a must and should be part of your ongoing routine to help keep skin toned. There are amazing 'face lift' massage techniques to help keep your skin working. The next step on from that would be CACI microcurrent facials, which target muscles to help lift the skin. These can be done in a course but can also be added in as part of tailored facials. Viora Reaction or Endymed glow radio frequency treatments work by stimulating collagen to lift and contour the skin. One of the stronger treatments used to target lax skin is Ultherapy, which uses ultrasound technology. This is usually carried out by a doctor or nurse. For both this and radio frequency, it will take about three months to see results.

The LED machine expert

Emily Byrne, Clinical Trainer from Tekno Surgical, distributor of Dermalux, explains how the LED machine works.

Dermalux LED uses clinical proven 'narrowband' wavelengths at the optimised intensity (power) and dose (time delivery) to enable photobiomodulation, the change to the targeted cells and skin tissue that light can trigger. Narrowband means that the wavelengths that Dermalux use are pure and laser-like without producing heat, and very specific. The table below shows the actions that the different types of Dermalux wavelengths perform on various skin conditions.

Wavelength	Power	Actions
The Resolve wavelength	Blue at 415nm (nanometres)	Specifically targets P. acnes bacteria (the acne-causing bacteria) to neutralise it
The Rejuvenate wavelength	Red at 633nm	Specifically targets the mitochondria of all cells, in this case reactivating fibroblast cells and promoting the growth of new collagen, elastin and hyaluronic acid production Stimulates blood and lymph circulation
The Regenerate wavelength	Near infrared (NIR) at 830nm	Like red, activates the mitochondria Anti-inflammatory, used to reduce inflammation in those with rosacea, acne, eczema, psoriasis and dermatitis Reduces inflammation and assists in tackling ageing Tyrosinase inhibitor to help control hyperpigmentation Stimulates TGF beta 3 to promote the generation of type 1 collagen

Light wavelengths are measured in nanometres (nm) and the wavelengths (opposite page) are the three most clinically proven wavelengths within the scientific community to target and address specific skin concerns.

Light works by targeting chromophores. For example, P. acne is a chromophore for blue light at 415nm (i.e. this kind of light will target acne). When these wavelengths are delivered and assume that the chromophore is present, they will trigger a response.

The first law of photobiology is that light must be absorbed to activate a cellular response. No absorption equals no reaction. So, we match the wavelength to target the chromophore (P. acnes, fibroblast cell and so on) and then deliver enough photon energy to reach the target. The energy of the device is thus vital!

Dermalux protocols are incredibly specific and based on scientific evidence and clinical trials, and our machines can deliver 1 wavelength at a time or all 3 concurrently without compromise due to the differing chromophores at different depths.

Regulations in Beauty Therapy

I have always felt the need for regulation within beauty therapy as a field, and I am proud to say that both Margaret O'Rourke Doherty (IMAGE Skillnet, HABIC) and Millie Kendall MBE (CEO of the British Beauty Council) are dedicated to making this a reality, in Ireland and the UK respectively.

The industry expert

Margaret O'Rourke Doherty is the founder and network manager of IMAGE Skillnet, a not-for-profit organisation that works to support the hair and beauty sector in Ireland, and the CEO of HABIC, the Hair and Beauty Industry Confederation. She is one of the key figures working towards better defined standards for those working in the beauty industry in Ireland.

Can you explain to us how standards within the beauty industry in Ireland work?

Until recently there were no defined European or national standards within the beauty industry, nor were there regulations with regard to skin, beauty therapy, hairdressing or any of the disciplines that are commonly associated as part of this industry. Additionally, the Health and Safety Authority implements legislation on health, safety and welfare in the workplace and the handling and usage of various chemical components. As it stands, almost anyone who wishes to do so can open and carry out treatments on clients – the only barrier is gaining public liability and treatment risk insurance.

In Ireland, for the most part, there are excellent operational procedures in salons that are delivered to the highest quality amongst industry professionals. However, like everything in life, there are variants in the level of professional knowledge, experience, quality and service delivered to the consumer.

In the absence of a defined standard or regulation, the industry has taken its cues relating to standards from the various education bodies. For years, professionals underwent high-quality, prolonged and intense training prior to entering the industry. This training gave the therapist in-depth knowledge which they continually added to over the course of their career. However, in recent times it is becoming more evident that a small minority of industry providers have not had in-depth core education, and are therefore left with significant gaps in their knowledge.

The majority of professionals nationally have upheld a very high standard of practice, but not all therapists or professionals are equal, nor are the professional qualifications they hold. It is essential for the safety of the consumer that the client can openly ask about the qualifications of the therapist that they will be treated by, especially as we move towards more aggressive treatments becoming the norm in the industry.

In October 2019, after years of work and engagement with the industry, the National Standards Authority of Ireland (NSAI) published the first European Standard for Beauty Salon Services, I.S. EN 17226, which sets out the requirements and recommendations for the provision of service in beauty salons. For now, this standard is voluntary and each salon can work towards the adoption of these standards. The Hair and Beauty Industry Confederation (HABIC) warmly welcomes this new EU Beauty Salon Standard and actively encourages salons and therapists to engage with this standard. Professional engagement with the standard will help ensure consistency of services nationally, protect the consumer and therapist, and raise the reputation of the industry.

CEO of the British Beauty Council

Millie Kendall MBE is the CEO of the British Beauty Council, and one half of iconic makeup brand Ruby & Millie. The British Beauty Council is a not-for-profit organisation that works to open channels of communication between the lucrative British beauty sector and the government, pushing for recognition and for better standards for consumers. We had a virtual sit-down and Millie provided lots of expert insight and information.

What base qualification do you feel a Botox practitioner should have?
In the industry, there is a big divide on whether it should be a doctor or a therapist. I think a lot of therapists would want to do it because it brings in money, and they have the demand from clients. However, there are horror stories and, to me, it's a medical procedure. I wouldn't want to have something like that done by somebody who isn't a doctor.

My concern is that the end user or the client may be aware that it's an invasive treatment, but they may not know that there are many adverse reactions that can happen …

Of course, and I'm more open to therapists giving this type of treatment when they are working in multi-disciplinary environments, for example if there are doctors on hand.

I believe that it's a special talent that should be reserved for few, not many, and I think that the consumer assumes that therapists' qualifications automatically include neurotoxins and injectables – I don't think they're aware that therapists aren't regulated.

I'm commonly asked if I perform Botox or fillers, and it's scary to realise that consumers aren't aware that these treatments aren't well regulated. IPL and laser and that tier of treatments, a tier 'below' Botox and injectables, is a whole new sector that has come to life. Do you believe this will always live underneath the beauty realm?

In the UK, you have to have completed the highest level (Level 7) for needling and laser. As part of my job at the British Beauty Council – I'm sort of responsible for the entire beauty industry here, in a way – there's a lot of detail I've learned over the past two years. One of the things I originally didn't understand was the different qualifications and what type of level you got for that within the beauty sector. I wouldn't have known to ask my therapist what level of qualification they had – you can go to Level 4, or Level 7, or stop anywhere in between – and I've been involved in the beauty sector since I was thirteen. If I didn't know to ask, I can imagine a lot of other people don't know.

For treatments like dermablading [a treatment involving a medical-grade blade to very gently 'shave' the surface of the skin, removing dead skin cells and fine hairs] *and microblading* [a form of semi-permanent tattooing, often used on the eyebrows] – *I would want a therapist who I know has the adequate training.*

We don't promote and certainly don't talk enough about training and qualifications, and because of this, consumers don't particularly understand whether or not the therapist has the correct qualifications for a procedure. I think the whole system is flawed because it's so complicated.

Is the education and awareness piece the largest piece you're trying to tackle – so that the consumer can make their own decisions?

We're [the British Beauty Council] *definitely a consumer-facing organisation, and I feel the lack of education and awareness within the industry is where we let the consumer down. Our reputation is heavily based on the information that the industry doesn't provide to the consumer.*

How can we raise awareness, in the UK or Ireland, so that the consumer can become more empowered? How do you envisage them having that mass market awareness of what the sector is and involves?

We have to look at the sector in general – what's really important about beauty and the direction it's moving in, particularly with the power of the internet, is that it's very consumer-driven. Brands of the future, the hugely successful brands, such as Glossier, are successful because they are consumer-driven.

Brands have to look at market trends – where is this going? If it's being led by the consumer, should we not be listening to what the consumer is asking for? Consumers are asking us for transparency, sustainability and efficacy. So in order to keep up with trends, we need to be on top of it, even though in general we are often lagging behind. They are going to start asking for transparency, and we need to be ready for this.

I feel that there is some disjointedness between the therapist, the brand and then the consumer – what we're all trying to do ultimately is tie the three together but more so focus on the consumer.

I think after world events like the Covid 19 pandemic in 2020, people will go back into salons and vote with their feet. If they walk into a salon where they don't have the appropriate equipment and the treatments are not carried out well hygienically and professionally, they will not come back, because there's a risk to their health.

You've always had a fascination with brands – this is the last lagging piece, tying brand to consumer and vice versa.

You need to move fast, think on your feet, and ask what the perception is. My dad's a hairdresser so I understand the service side of it fairly well, but when I used to have a shop, I used to stand outside the front door and watch what it looked like from the outside. What's the perception of it? Does it look tatty? Does it look clean enough? What's the consumer's perception of my business? At the end of the day, it's a business – you're marketing your services. I think we're going to have to get used to a lot of changes. But I think that if you were transparent and you had a sign on your salon window that said 'I have completed Level 7', which is the highest level in beauty therapy training in the UK, I believe the consumer would respond to that. If I went into a salon and I had the choice of four therapists, I would want to pick them based on the level of qualifications they've received!

I don't think we're transparent enough with levels of qualifications.

Why is this so important to you personally and professionally? Why have you taken on such a massive role that is part of everything involved in the sector?

The most personal thing to me was the fact that in 2007, I was awarded an MBE. It was quite a monumental moment and it came as a bit of a surprise, but unfortunately there can be a flippant kind of attitude towards the beauty industry – mostly men, but not just men. If I'm sitting at a dinner party, and I say I work in the beauty industry, they sort of look at me and then turn to speak to someone who they perceive is more intelligent.

I think I just got sick of it. I know so many clever people in this industry, some people who came through finance, some came from legal ... It's not necessarily just about the services themselves.

One of the things we're trying to do is lobby government to move hairdressers into the highly skilled workers' category. Currently, we're considered labourers.

How do you stop that ignorance from others?

There are several things: there is good PR, there's increased standards within the industry which is a long road but the focus and prioritisation of safety protocols and hygiene standards as a result of the Covid 19 pandemic will, in ten months, get us to a place which might have otherwise taken ten years because people are going to have to pull their socks up. Equally, education is important – I mean promoting careers to those between the ages of 13 and 16 and equally looking at higher education courses. For example, L'Oréal has just put together a bachelor's degree in hairdressing.

There are careers within the beauty industry that are outside of services that could add to the overall image of beauty, but having said that, we have to be conscious not to downgrade the services side of the industry. As we've seen during this situation, the thing people want the most is their eyebrows tweezed and their hair coloured. However vacuous you like to think it is, it's actually really important for people's mental wellbeing.

If you were to think ahead about ten years, what would you like the future of our sector to look like?

More respect for the services side of our industry. I'd like to see degrees in different elements – beauty communication, beauty buying, beauty education – you should be able to have a degree in being a beauty educator.

I'd like to see a diversity in education: I'd like to see all courses in the UK cover dark skin and dark hair; at the moment I feel the courses are very white-centric, I think that's unacceptable.

I also want to see a slowdown of products being developed and launched; I'd like to see good NPD [new product development]. When I was younger, we had seasonal products being launched, now something is launched every five minutes and it is adding to our poor reputation in terms of sustainability and that sucks, that's not good for us at all.

The last point would be to understand how your MBE came about, what it was awarded for, and how it feels to represent the sector.

There are ways of getting them, and I guess you must be recommended. I don't know who recommended me, but I have a suspicion that it was Cherie Blair because she called up and asked me to do her makeup. I'm not a makeup artist, but I had a brand, so she assumed that was something I could do. I found out about this just before I had my daughter; I had my daughter, and then I had to wait until January to hear if I was included.

They send you a letter before that says you might have got it. Obviously, I had told everyone and then read the fine print where it says please do not tell anyone. My mum was very unwell at the time, so I think she thought she was in an episode of The Crown, *my dad flew in from LA. It was incredibly emotional, actually, and I didn't expect it to be. I just didn't get it; I don't think I understood it at all. I don't think you quite understand it until it happens and then you think 'okay, I get it now'.*

Do they tell you why you deserve it?
They say it's for services to the cosmetics industry, and they just go Ruby Hammer and Millicent Kendall. It was so nerve-wracking, but all I cared about was not falling over. I had high shoes on, and the carpet was very slippery. I felt like I moon-walked the whole way towards the Queen. It was terrible, it was awful; it was okay, but quite embarrassing. All I remember was that she smelled really good, she smelled of roses. I am proud of it, but equally, it's a bit daunting sometimes. I just swear and put everyone at ease.

The pharmacist

I invited a pharmacist to give us an insight into her role in terms of skincare. Pharmacists are vital and with Skingredients, we work alongside so many and hold all in esteem. I have worked closely alongside Oonagh O'Hagan, owner and managing director of the Meaghers Pharmacy Group in Dublin, and she has been, 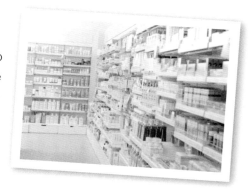 first and foremost, a mentor, an inspiration and a person I always feel will give accurate, succinct and valuable advice. She is a keen advocate of education and really builds a community with her customers. I wanted to learn her view on skincare from her perspective.

What role do you think pharmacists play in the treatment of customers' skin conditions?
Pharmacists are uniquely placed in that we can advise and offer consultations to our customers who may be in need of expert advice around the treatment

and prevention of skin conditions. For example, some customers may visit us with prescriptions for potentially photo-sensitising medications, such as immunosuppressants, and we know that their medication may lead to a heightened sensitivity of their skin to sunlight. We can advise them on how to proactively prevent such conditions from arising, how to use a broad-spectrum SPF product and to reapply throughout the day. Other medications, such as Roaccutane, may lead to excessive dryness in the skin and we can proactively recommend intense emollients that will prevent their skin from becoming dehydrated in the first instance. So pharmacists play a unique role not only in the treatment of skin conditions but often in the prevention of such conditions emerging.

Customers may visit us with a physical flare-up of their skin, such as an aggressive breakout of acne. As well as being in physical pain, customers can be incredibly self-conscious or even embarrassed and there often may be a knock-on effect on their confidence and self-esteem. Because of this, our approach is always one of empathy and understanding, giving our customers the advice and reassurance they need, whilst asking questions about their lifestyle, their diet, stress and other factors with an aim at getting to the root of the flare-up, and then providing advice tailored to each individual. From a thorough consultation, we can see the bigger picture and can provide not only skincare products but often other advice on dietary changes or supplements that can support a more speedy recovery, together with tips on lifestyle changes that can help.

When it comes to skincare, it's important that we as pharmacists are fully trained to provide qualified advice on skin concerns. Many customers present to us perhaps looking for a specific product that they've heard recommended by a friend or an influencer. Although it may be an effective product for their friend, sister or an influencer, it won't always be right for them so we try to ensure that if they are looking to purchase a specific product, they know what ingredients it contains, who it is beneficial for, and if it will actually suit their skin. Very often, we find that the product they believe they need is quite simply unsuitable for their skin type and would only lead to further aggravation of the particular concern that they are attempting to rectify. We find that this continuous education is what helps our customers understand their own skin type and make more qualified choices on what ingredients they actually need to address their particular concern. We will try to help them to find what will work best for their skin. We very often have customers come in with quite serious damage and even burns to their skin after using retinoids or alpha-hydroxy acids without having received advice first, and fortunately, with our qualification, we're in a position where we can provide expert advice on what can help them to deal with the consequences and treat the damage that may have been caused.

If a customer has tried over-the-counter options for their skin concerns for a period of time and haven't seen improvement, we'll refer to a GP, a dermatologist, or a GP that we know has a special interest in dermatology or skin. We can signpost customers to get the advice they need from the most appropriate healthcare provider, be that their GP or another specialist who can help them find the solutions they need.

When it comes to dietary and nutritional concerns, we're highly trained and keep abreast of the cutting-edge research in supplements, and we only stock reputable high-quality brands which are backed by clinical research. We will often recommend, for example, the probiotic Symprove, for those looking to take care of their gut health but also for many inflammatory skin conditions. Research shows that inflammatory bowel conditions are linked to an imbalance in your microbiome and we can now see that looking after your microbiome has so many other health benefits. Many customers report a positive impact on inflammatory conditions such as psoriasis, eczema and rosacea when taking Symprove. If we feel that a skin condition could be linked to poor diet or a particular lifestyle, we can recommend a range of supplements for given concerns, be these acne breakouts or dehydrated, ageing skin. We also refer many customers to dietitians who can take a look at their overall diet and recommend positive change that can make real and lasting differences to many skin concerns. As a pharmacist, I firmly believe that we must always treat the skin from within and in synergy with a bespoke skincare routine. We see many more positive and long-lasting changes when we take this multi-pronged approach to the particular skin concern, be that acne, rosacea, dehydration or to slow down the ageing process of the skin.

At Meaghers, we see our role as pharmacists as educators in the importance of good skin health. As healthcare professionals, our pharmacists are fully trained to take a holistic view of our customers' overall health and wellbeing as part of a multi-faceted approach to the recommendation of a suitable skincare routine.

The GP

The GP is a central figure in the jigsaw, because they are often the first port of call and also perform the role of a connector, pulling the network of experts together as needed on their patient's behalf.

Dr Olga is our resident nerdie GP, with a special interest in dermatology: those within the Nerd Network who our team feel may benefit from medical advice are referred to Dr Olga. Prior to the appointment, each Nerd Networker completes a medical evaluation form that allows Dr Olga to be prepared and to have everything she needs to safely prescribe medication for them, if that is what she feels is best. So she's an important skincare ally to The Skin Nerd!

A GP visit can be the single most important step in managing skin concerns. It is an unbiased and objective service and can also help you get access to other experts/services you might need.

What is the role of the GP in skincare?

Consultations relating to skin disorders account for approximately 20 per cent of day-to-day GP presentations. In my own daily practice, I encounter a multitude of skin-related problems every day, ranging from minor to more severe, and including males and females of all age profiles, from infancy through to old age. It is no surprise that skin function (and dysfunction) are at the forefront of primary care medicine. Covering an average of 2 square metres and weighing in at around 3.6 kilograms for adults, the skin is the body's largest and heaviest organ. An average square inch of skin contains a staggering 650 sweat glands, 20 blood vessels and more than 1,000 nerve endings ... quite impressive when you consider that skin is only a few millimetres thick. Skin is an amazingly versatile organ with a plethora of functions that are vital to human life. We all visit our GP when we are feeling acutely unwell and for management of chronic medical conditions. Equally, we must keep in mind that our skin is an organ too and should be cared for and treated with the same respect that we lend to the rest of our bodies.

'Skin is in', as they say, and as a GP I have certainly seen an increase in skin presentations to primary care both for medical and cosmetic reasons. I am always delighted to see people who are keen to invest in their skin health. Common skin presentations to GP include: skin rashes, discolouration/ pigmentation, lumps/bumps/lesions, acne, rosacea, psoriasis, eczema, and allergy ... to name a few! While many of these presentations are specific to the skin itself, some may be a sign of a more serious underlying condition. It is imperative that these skin/systemic problems are correctly identified and managed appropriately. All too often these days 'Doctor Google' is consulted and relied upon for a diagnosis and management plan. This can lead to misinformation, incorrect diagnoses, and ineffective or even harmful treatments.

Your GP should be your first port of call for accurate medical information regarding skin conditions. He or she can offer you unbiased, evidence-based, reliable advice and guide you along your skincare journey. While skin health and minor skin ailments may be managed with a skincare regime that is tailored to your individual needs, some skin problems and associated conditions require medical management. While many of these skin conditions can be treated within general practice, the 'gate-keeper' role of the GP is such that appropriate referral of complex cases to tertiary care (i.e. to a consultant dermatologist or other medical consultant) can also be arranged. Equally, a referral to a dietitian or aesthetic practitioner may be most appropriate, and again this can be guided by your GP.

How does your GP provide a holistic, multi-faceted approach in skincare?

The condition and appearance of our skin is the cumulative effect of intrinsic and extrinsic factors. Our intrinsic genetics determining skin type and biological ageing cannot be altered, but many other skin changes and premature skin ageing are heavily influenced by external factors, including our daily habits and lifestyle.

Your GP can play a key role in guiding and improving your lifestyle choices and promoting better skin health alongside overall improvements in wellbeing. Advice, and medical management where appropriate relating to nutrition, smoking cessation, sleep hygiene and stress reduction, can all be covered as part of the GP consultation. We GPs understand that initiating lifestyle changes in any area of concern can be hugely challenging and fraught with difficulty, and can offer you support and information to lessen the load of this journey. Complementary medical treatments may be utilised in some instances for a multi-faceted approach to wellbeing. 'Talk to your GP' is something we hear time and time again. A simple first step that really does work.

Perhaps the most important role of the GP in the skin expert jigsaw is to correctly identify the exact nature of the problem in the first instance. The 'what is it, Doctor?' question, if you will. This is especially important when it comes to skin lesions (skin or a growth that doesn't look the same as the skin around it) – differentiating benign lesions from potentially dangerous malignant lesions and treating them appropriately. In the case of melanoma skin cancer, for example, early diagnosis and referral for specialist treatment can be life-saving.

Other skin problems necessitating medical management include acne, rosacea, psoriasis and eczema. Hormonal changes of puberty and menopause can contribute, and thus a thorough medical history, often in conjunction with blood tests, will help your GP in their investigative process. Mild and moderate cases of the above can be well managed within general practice using a combination of topical and oral treatments, alongside lifestyle measures. In severe cases, a referral to a consultant dermatologist may be warranted for advanced treatments, including immunotherapies.

Aesthetic dermatology is becoming more and more common in general practice, with many GPs now equipped to advise on anti-ageing skincare, correction of skin texture and pigmentation, or even perform injectable anti-ageing therapies.

A visit to your GP is an important first step for skin and related issues, especially those of a moderate or severe nature. Information is power. From there your skin journey can begin.

The cosmetic doctor

Another highly regarded skin specialist is Dr Katherine Mulrooney of the Dr Mulrooney Clinic, a cosmetic doctor. A cosmetic doctor is one who specialises in non-surgical cosmetic treatments and procedures. I sat alongside the Mulrooneys, Dr Katherine and her sister, Dr Jane, on a panel some years ago and beyond their pure elegance, there was passion and dedication to an art, a refined and articulate art – their work is tasteful and unnoticeable, which is the desired effect for many. They are also fellow skincare formulators with their own organic seaweed-based skincare range, SEAVITE – they truly understand the diversity of the skincare sector as a whole. I invited Dr Katherine to give us her expert advice on fillers, which are becoming more popular within the beauty industry.

Tell me all you know about fillers.

Filler is made from pure cross-linked hyaluronic acid gel that mimics your own natural hyaluronic acid, which gives plumpness to your skin. Hyaluronic acid can hold 100 times its weight in water, which allows it to occupy large volumes relative to its mass. The hyaluronic acid used in fillers is derived from either the combs of rooster birds or from the synthetic fermentation of Staphylococcus equine bacterium! The bacterial-derived hyaluronic acid tends to be purer, more viscous and less likely to cause an allergy than the bird-derived version and hence is more commonly used. And this form is longer-lasting due to the cross-linking agent.

Clinically approved fillers in Europe include Belotero (from MERZ Pharmaceuticals), Juvéderm (from Allergan) and Restylane (Q-Med), with many more coming to the market year on year. The product must carry a CE mark of approval as fillers are considered a medical device. In practice, fillers are used to treat the five As:

* *Ageing skin – from the age of about 25 years onwards, the skin begins to lose its natural hyaluronic acid and collagen, making it less plump and more prone to fine lines and wrinkles.*
* *Atrophic (skin thinning) scars, e.g. pitted acne scarring.*

* Atrophic of the skin, e.g. due to chronic overuse of steroids, burns or traumas.
* Asymmetry – natural, post-operative or post-trauma.
* Augmentation – primarily lips and cheeks.

The most popular use of filler at the Dr Mulrooney Clinic is to replace lost volume on the face, most notably the nasolabial lines (from the corners of the nose to the mouth), perioral lines, smoker's lines, cheeks, lips and temple area and the treatment of acne scarring post-resurfacing laser, such as Fraxel, to correct facial asymmetry and soften pitted acne scarring.

A filler procedure takes approximately one hour. The patient is numbed with numbing cream for 30 minutes, the face is then cleaned, sterilised, marked and finally injected. Post-injection, ice packs are applied for a minimum of 15 minutes to minimise swelling. It is advised not to wear any makeup or any moisturiser/cosmetics for the rest of the day to avoid contamination of the fresh injection sites.

Afterwards the area is red and swollen for two to three hours. Bruising can occur and can last for seven to ten days. We advise patients to start taking arnica tablets and stop alcohol, aspirin, anti-inflammatories and fish oils for five days before the treatment in order to minimise the risk of bruising.

Fillers work very well with botulinum toxin (Botox) injections and laser for optimal facial rejuvenation. We call this 'Triple Therapy'. First, we use botulinum toxin to lift and soften expression lines, followed by laser to improve skin texture, tone and radiance, and finally we use filler to replace lost volume on the face. This gives a very natural and balanced facial rejuvenation.

Possible unwanted side-effects of fillers include:
* swelling and bruising at the site of the injection
* infection at the site of injection
* inflammatory responses
* hypersensitivity reactions
* nodule or granuloma formation (structures formed as a result of inflammation)

* *vascular occlusion (blood vessel blockage) and tissue necrosis.*

Contraindications/reasons not to choose fillers:
* *pregnancy and breastfeeding*
* *infection at the proposed injection site, e.g. herpes simplex*
* *known hypersensitivity to hyaluronic acid or lidocaine*
* *granuloma annulare (common condition consisting of raised discoloured areas on the skin)*
* *sarcoidosis (an inflammatory disease)*
* *lupus*

The antidote 'hyaluronidase' can be used to dissolve unwanted hyaluronic acid filler; however, it is worth noting this dissolves both natural and injected hyaluronic acid, so it is best avoided.

The cosmetic surgeon

Mr Kambiz Golchin is held in high esteem and comes highly recommended, and his set-up in the Beacon is second to none. He is considered a pioneer and sits on many panels and advisory boards because of this. He has been generous with his time in an advisory capacity with regard to Skingredients. He is a gentleman and excellent at his job.

How do you feel plastic surgeons can work alongside other professionals such as GPs, cosmetic doctors, dermatologists and skin therapists?
Plastic and cosmetic surgeons are well used to working in a team. Indeed, this is such an integral part of our training that it is almost second nature to us. We all know that the best outcome is achieved by a multidisciplinary approach, and I think there has been a shift from the patient's perspective. With the abundance of information available on aesthetics on the internet and social media, the patients are in the driving seat and are choosing multiple practitioners and

procedures. This makes it imperative for all of the professionals to work together closely in the interest of the patient.

Can you give an example or two of how a client may be referred to a plastic surgeon, or how (or what) you would refer to any of the mentioned professionals, including GPs, dermatologists or skin therapists?

A good example is a typical patient with excessive sun damage, pigmentation, volume loss and wrinkles who has been receiving skin treatments by a skin therapist and/or dermatologist and is looking for better results. Such a patient could ultimately be suitable for plastic surgery such as fat grafting and facelift, or more likely nowadays they would be offered the latest volume replacement treatments such as stem cell fat grafting or laser resurfacing.

How can one work to improve scarring following cosmetic procedures in terms of skincare, diet and general care?

Improving scarring is one of the main principles of all cosmetic procedures. The skill of the surgeon is an important factor. However, there are lots of other factors which can be controlled by the individual. From a dietary point of view, a well-balanced diet with an emphasis on protein intake, vitamin C and zinc is important. Avoiding smoking and drinking an excessive amount of alcohol is also important. There is good evidence that optimising skin with a good skincare routine can improve the overall aesthetic results, and this can involve the use of potent antioxidants, retinols, medical-grade facials, and of course, regular use of SPF.

The dermatologist

The dermatologist is a key piece in the expert jigsaw puzzle and Dr Cal Condon is held in high esteem – a consummate professional and a true intellectual. However, what struck me upon meeting him was his empathy, compassion and real human desire to assist his patients. The importance of treating illnesses that others are unable to can't be measured. Qualified individuals like Dr Cal Condon dedicate years to one subject so that they can address these topics and concerns. The respect I have for this profession is endless. I'm honoured to include a contribution from Dr Condon in the book and delighted that we share the same multi-disciplinary approach to skincare.

Can you give us an insight into the work and practices of a dermatologist?

Dermatology is a medical subspecialty and GPs and dermatologists are best placed to advise and manage diseases of the skin. It is my view that in order to diagnose skin disease, it is first essential to know what diseases exist and to be able to differentiate between them. A case in point would be the angry red face that can occur in association with rosacea, but also in seborrheic dermatitis, demodex folliculitis, psoriasis, irritant dermatitis, allergic dermatitis or photo dermatitis, as part of an underlying medical condition such as lupus, or as a manifestation of internal cancer such as dermatomyositis, and many others.

In the current commercial world, where people are extremely concerned over appearance, there is a second level of skincare where the skin is not diseased but where all treatments and therapies are directed towards improving the appearance. This can take the form of dietary modifications, skincare recommendations and physical therapies. Many of these therapies have traditionally been undertaken in the beauty sector, but over the last one to two decades there has been something of a collision between the two sectors. This is largely due to commercial considerations and the advent of new physical therapies, such as laser, IPL and radiofrequency treatments.

In some areas, such as laser hair removal, therapies have moved from dermatologists to salons as the technology becomes safer and demand has increased. Unfortunately, commercial investors have flooded the market and, in many instances, salons endeavour to treat skin disease or undertake procedures that may have significant side-effects, such as filler injections and invasive laser treatments. It is my opinion that no one should undertake a procedure that has significant side-effects if they are not trained to deal with them.

Skin therapists provide physical therapies and skincare, makeup and cosmetic camouflage advice, and ideally are concerned with management and optimal presentation of non-diseased skin. I think it is unfortunate that there is not more cross-cooperation between these groups as this is, I think, the pathway to the best patient care.

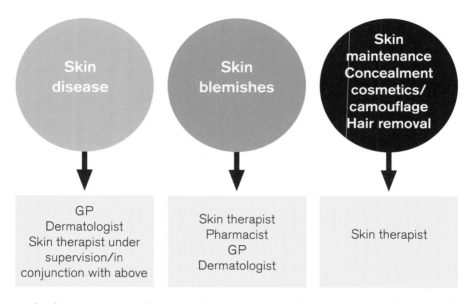

In the past, cosmetic corrections were considered the area of the plastic surgeon, skin disease the area of the dermatologist and more immediate but temporary beauty treatments the area of the salon beautician. Over the last two decades, these demarcations have blurred considerably. Many dermatologists now do corrective surgical procedures, plastic surgeons use lasers and other technology to treat skin disease, and beauticians use lasers and inject fillers. All three dispense or recommend cosmeceuticals and other anti-ageing or remedial products. In a perfect world, all three groups would work together as a team which might also include a dietitian or nutritionist.

My list above is an opinion as to how patients might flow within such a grouping, with the doctors looking after active skin disease and the nurse practitioner or skin therapist providing a more hands-on approach to care and the delivery of that care. In such a scenario, the doctor would diagnose and set out a treatment plan. Where appropriate, medical, surgical or laser interventions would take place first that would be partly or wholly carried out by the doctor, nurse or other specialist practitioner. Skin problems not associated with a skin disease or those requiring camouflage or temporary correction (skincare product advice and usage, application of makeup or dyes, hair removal, nutritional advice, exfoliation procedures, etc.) would fall under the remit of the skin therapist. This model would, in my opinion, allow patients to access the best available care. Take an example of a patient who was burnt on the scalp: one would first treat the burn, then try to minimise the scarring. After this the patient might benefit from laser therapy, advice on cosmetic camouflage and fitting for a hair piece or wig. Each step is important but the combination gives the best possible result for the patient.

What treatments are available for acne?

Acne is an extremely common chronic inflammatory disease that can range from congested pores and a couple of pimples to an extensive, painful, scarring disease that can result in life-long disfigurement. For milder disease, most sufferers will try easily available over-the-counter products before seeking medical advice. Many of the traditional first-line therapies can irritate the skin and this has led to the emergence of so-called cosmeceuticals (cosmetic meets pharmaceutical – or products containing active ingredients). There is a growing amount of research being done on cosmeceuticals and their mechanisms of action in treating acne. These products can be used as monotherapy or in combination with medical treatment and are broadly grouped into products that reduce oil production (topical antioxidants and niacinamide), agents targeting abnormal

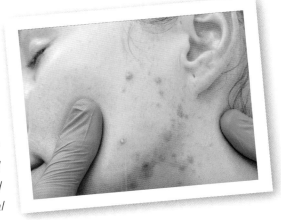

keratinisation and sticky skin (salicylic acid, alpha-hydroxy acids, retinol-based products and linoleic acid), agents targeting Propionibacterium acnes (lauric acid) and anti-inflammatory agents (nicotinamide [commonly known as niacinamide], alpha-linolenic acid and zinc salts). Despite the advances in understanding these cosmetic ingredients, there still remains a lack of controlled studies in this area.

What is the most common prescription for acne?

Antibiotics, both topical and oral. This is odd given that acne is a hormonal-induced skin disease of excess oil production. Antibiotics treat the effects, not the cause, and are, at best, a modest treatment. Roaccutane (isotretinoin) and topical retinoids are far more effective but are associated with significant side-effects. Spironolactone and the oral contraceptive pill are usually well-tolerated in females and are effective.

Combination therapies emerging for acne include low-dosage Roaccutane and laser, which treats the acne and the scarring simultaneously, but this does extend the duration of therapy. Notably, pregnancy must be avoided during Roaccutane treatment due to the risk of birth defects.

Photodynamic therapy is another area that shows promise. The basic principle is that a drug, applied to the skin, can be concentrated in the sebaceous gland. This drug is then activated using a light or laser source which in turn damages the sebaceous gland, thereby reducing oil production and alleviating acne.

In my experience, dietary manipulation is of very limited value in acne management. Dairy products, peanuts and foods high in glucose are best avoided, but restriction alone rarely produces significant improvement.

Glycolic acid, alpha-hydroxy acid and salicylic acid are all useful in treating acne, but are all a little irritating on the skin. Hyaluronic acid is less irritating and less studied but is certainly useful in patients who are irritated by the other products. SPF and antioxidants are a recommended and positive addition to any skin regimen and help prevent sun damage and photo-ageing. Their role as active agents in treating or preventing acne is unproven but, and it is an *important but, acne treatments can irritate the skin and irritated skin is more susceptible to sun damage than non-irritated skin: as such I believe that they are an important part of an acne skin regimen.*

Tell us about rosacea

Rosacea is an unusual disease. The cause is unknown but the most recent research suggests that it is a disorder of the skin microbiome. This imbalance results in the release of inflammatory agents that mediate redness, new blood vessel formation and inflammatory papules. Dietary manipulations can have a significant effect on rosacea but appear to vary between individuals. Topical therapies to reduce the numbers of Demodex mites (a type of mite that lives on the skin, believed to be linked to rosacea), and oral or topical antibiotics (thought to act as anti-inflammatories) are usually very effective, but maintenance therapy is usually required. Laser and IPL can greatly reduce the redness and flushing, as can some drugs, such as beta blockers. Interestingly, Roaccutane, in low dose, can be very effective and this is presumed to be secondary to alterations in the skin oil content. These alterations change the microenvironment of the skin and reduce the tendency of the microbiome to become imbalanced.

Patients suffering from rosacea tend to have sensitive skin, which can be easily irritated by certain skincare ingredients, including alpha-hydroxy and beta-hydroxy acids, retinol and alcohol. Skincare advice is very important for this group of patients and includes gentle washing, avoiding abrasive scrubs, as well as limiting chemicals and non-natural ingredients to help reduce the likelihood of rosacea flare-ups. The American Academy of Dermatology emphasises the importance of moisturising the skin every day, which can help reduce irritation as well as dryness. Using a rosacea-friendly moisturiser or barrier repair cream twice a day has been proven to improve patient comfort

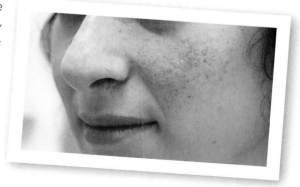

levels, as well as peeling, roughness and other common rosacea symptoms. Fragrance-free products containing antioxidants – green tea, niacinamides, and ceramides – can decrease redness and improve the skin's barrier. Natural calming ingredients like cucumber and chamomile extract can also reduce redness and irritation as can turmeric-containing creams, which have anti-inflammatory products that can help with flare-ups.

Processed foods, chemicals and high-sugar foods are known to cause systemic inflammation, which can promote the inflammatory processes of the skin and redness commonly associated with rosacea. One of the primary strategies for managing the condition is improving dietary choices; this includes eliminating triggers and adding nutritious foods. In addition, patients should be advised to avoid dietary triggers that can aggravate rosacea, such as eliminating or limiting alcohol and caffeine consumption, hot showers, and spicy foods. Patients who may not be aware of their individual dietary triggers should be urged to keep a food diary to determine exact food, beverage and spice reactions.

What about psoriasis?

Psoriasis has now clearly been shown to be a disorder of the innate immune system that is genetically mediated. It is a disease, it is treatable and it should remain in the hands of the specialists. (This also applies for acne and rosacea, although there is obviously more of a role for alternative therapies with these conditions particularly where the disease is mild and medications might not be appropriate.)

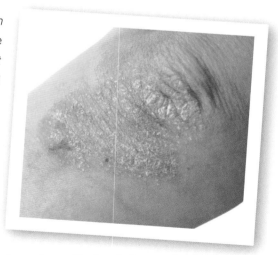

Do you think most people know how to self-check for moles?

No, no, no, unfortunately! The ABCDE of self-exam (asymmetry, border, colours, diameter and evolution) and the ugly duckling sign (melanoma will often stand out from the others, like an ugly duckling) are very useful and I advocate self-exams. I also recommend mole mapping with close-up digital dermoscopic imaging of irregular moles. However, even with these tools and more than 20 years' experience, I am regularly unsure.

Doctors and dermatologists remove large numbers of benign moles simply because diagnosis is so difficult. I regularly say to patients, 'It looks benign, but I'm not sure and if I'm wrong, the consequences are severe.' Removing a mole is simple, safe and will give certainty.

This is all fantastic advice from Dr Condon, but I was curious to know his stance on skin therapies as well. It was interesting to hear that he's a fan.

What are your thoughts on current concepts in rejuvenation and restoration?

Although the ageing process is entirely natural, it is associated with a number of undesirable effects, both from a medical and an aesthetic viewpoint. At my practice at Dermatology Matters, we strive to address all aspects of ageing skin both to reduce age-related skin diseases and cancers and, where possible, to combine treatments so as to also produce a more youthful and fresh appearance. Our goal is the restoration of what was lost. In terms of prevention, ultraviolet sunlight is one of the major causes of skin ageing and skin cancer. Daily sun protection using a high-quality sun block is an essential part of any skincare regimen. This is adequate for minimal exposure but SPF should be reapplied every two to three hours if exposed to more intense sunlight.

What about treatments for ageing?

Modalities (tools) used to correct or repair aged skin target more specific problems. Firstly, the skin is examined for any skin cancer or pre-cancerous changes and these are treated accordingly with surgery, cryosurgery, photodynamic therapy or topical chemotherapy. Then the skin is examined for evidence of non-cancerous sun damage, such as sun spots, thread veins and laxity. These blemishes can also be treated using a combination of therapies, *including IPL, Nd:YAG, Fraxel, Active FX and photodynamic therapy. Topical therapies can also be used although they are most effective at maintaining the improvements achieved with more potent therapy.*

What are your thoughts on IPL and laser therapies?

I am a big advocate for IPL and laser therapies. IPL stands for intense pulsed light, and it is a treatment used to treat hyperpigmentation, brown spots, thread veins and erythema and fine lines and wrinkles caused by sun damage. The results are rapid and the treatment is very well tolerated. Typically, three to five treatment sessions are needed. IPL treatments also improve skin texture through collagen stimulation, reduce pore size and temporarily reduce oiliness.

Fraxel is a non-invasive laser treatment that makes hundreds of thousands of microscopic holes in the skin. This softens and elevates scars and wrinkles and as the skin heals it tightens due to the production of new collagen and elastin within the dermis or deeper layer of the skin. Basically, it smooths wrinkles and scars, fades brown spots, and resurfaces your entire skin tone. Unlike ablative lasers, Fraxel is a fractional skin-resurfacing treatment, which means it only targets a fraction of the skin at a time. This means that after treatment the skin appears a little red and puffy, but there is no real downtime. The number of sessions required varies, but usually three to six sessions are required. Active FX is a more aggressive therapy, similar to Fraxel, but using a CO_2 laser as opposed to an Erbium glass laser. Active FX gives better results but is associated with greater post-procedure downtime, which typically lasts three to four days.

Skin laxity and collagen loss can be reversed using a combination of different modalities. IPL and Fraxel operate at a superficial level and are suitable for fine lines and wrinkles on the face, whereas the Nd:YAG laser and bipolar radiofrequency (Viora Reaction) operate at a deeper level and are more suited to the neck, forehead and deeper wrinkles.

Can you talk to us about the different types of skin cancer?

Skin cancer can be divided into two broad categories:

*   *Melanoma, which accounts for 4 per cent of all skin cancers*

* *Non-melanoma skin cancers, which account for 96 per cent of all skin cancers*
These two types of skin cancer behave very differently.

Melanoma Skin Cancer
Melanoma is a serious form of skin cancer. Finding melanoma at an early stage is crucial. Look for anything new, changing or unusual on both sun-exposed and sun-protected areas of the body. Melanomas commonly appear on the legs of women, while the number one place they develop on men is the trunk (torso). Keep in mind, though, that melanomas can arise anywhere on the skin, even in areas where the sun doesn't shine. Most moles, brown spots and growths on the skin are harmless – but not always. Go back to the ABCDEs and the ugly duckling sign [see page 239] to detect melanoma. Most normal moles on your body resemble one another, while melanomas stand out like ugly ducklings in comparison. This highlights the importance of not just checking for irregularities, but also comparing any suspicious spot to surrounding moles to determine whether it looks different than its neighbours.
* *Know the clinical features: anything new, changing or unusual.*
* *Prevention: sun avoidance or protection. Early detection: self-examination, medical examination.*

Non-melanoma skin cancer

Basal cell carcinoma
Basal cell carcinoma (BCC) is the most common form of skin cancer and the most common cancer in humans. BCCs arise from abnormal, uncontrolled growth of basal cells in the skin. Because BCCs grow slowly, most are curable and cause minimal damage if caught and treated early. Below are the warning signs for a BCC.
* *An open sore that does not heal, and may bleed, ooze or crust. The sore might persist for weeks, or appear to heal and then come back.*
* *A reddish patch or irritated area, on the face, chest, shoulder, arm or leg that may crust, itch, hurt or cause no discomfort.*

* A shiny bump or nodule that is pearly or clear, pink, red or white. The bump can also be tan, black or brown, especially in dark-skinned people, and can be mistaken for a normal mole.
* A small pink growth with a slightly raised, rolled edge and a crusted indentation in the centre that may develop tiny surface blood vessels over time.
* A scar-like area that is flat, white, yellow or waxy in colour. The skin appears shiny and taut, often with poorly defined borders.

Actinic keratosis:

An actinic keratosis is a rough, scaly patch on your skin that develops from years of exposure to the sun. A small percentage of lesions of this type can eventually become skin cancer.

* Clinical features: texture flat to slightly raised, scaly and/or rough
* Size: from a couple of millimetres up to 2cm in diameter
* Colour: may vary from skin-coloured to red, tan, pink or silvery
* Location: areas exposed to a lot of UV light such as the scalp, face, ears, lips, and the back of the hands and forearm.

Squamous cell carcinoma (SCC)

SCC occurs when DNA damage from exposure to ultraviolet radiation or other damaging agents triggers abnormal changes in the squamous cells in the epidermis. SCCs can appear as scaly red patches, open sores, rough, thickened or wart-like skin, or raised growths with a central depression. At times, SCCs may crust over, itch or bleed. The lesions most commonly arise in sun-exposed areas of the body.

SCC of the skin can develop anywhere on the body but is most often found on areas exposed to ultraviolet (UV) radiation like the face, lips, ears, scalp, shoulders, neck, back of the hands and forearms. SCCs can develop in scars, skin sores and other areas of skin injury. The skin around them typically shows signs of sun damage such as wrinkling, pigment changes and loss of elasticity. SCCs can appear as thick, rough, scaly patches that may crust or bleed. They can also resemble warts, or open sores that don't completely heal. Sometimes

SCCs show up as growths that are raised at the edges with a lower area in the centre that may bleed or itch.

* *Prevention: daily sun protection (slip on a shirt, slap on a hat, slop on the sunscreen).*
* *Early detection: medical examination of at-risk individuals and suspicious lesions, i.e. new, crusted or bleeding lesions on an at-risk site.*
* *Medical intervention: cryosurgery, surgical excision, laser ablation, topical chemotherapy, photodynamic therapy.*

Note from Jennifer:
The skin is an organ. Please don't dwell on the past, but ensure you use light protection now and in the future.

YOU

Yes, you! The last piece in the jigsaw. You are your skin's best advocate and protector; whatever choice you make when it comes to skincare, expert help or treatments, achieving better skin health is going to require ongoing work from you as well. You don't rock up at the dentist's twice a year and expect that to take care of your dental hygiene. No, you brush and floss daily as well. And the very same is true for your skin. All of the advice from our panel of experts is excellent and helpful and you might choose to follow some of it, but you can't hand over responsibility for your skin to anyone else. Seek guidance from the right expert and take comfort in knowing that there are many approaches to the health of this organ – so there will be a way that aligns with your needs and goals and provides real results.

The Tenth Nerdie Principle

Balance is Sacred

The bottom-line rule in skincare is: balance – equilibrium – homeostasis. This is a sacred principle from which all goodness flows. The ingredients you choose to put onto your skin must be balanced to address your skin concerns and deliver the results you want, but do so in a way that is gentle and also respectful of your skin's natural processes. My own preference is for ingredients that work together to encourage your skin's own abilities, gently nudging it to do what it's supposed to be doing. So, for example, I adore PrePro which very, very gently exfoliates with polyhydroxy acid, gives back, soothes and hydrates with the prebiotic-probiotic complex. When you have balance, you don't need the strong-arm tactics when you're using everything correctly. That's the fundamental approach of Skingredients and of all good skincare – be progressive and respectful, and results will ensue. Everything we recommend leads back to our motto: the skin is an organ, respect it accordingly. We do that by feeding it on the inside and taking care of it on the outside and on top - a careful balance that allows us to achieve skin health.

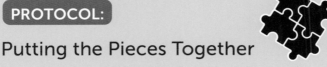

Putting the Pieces Together

Do you think that your skin concern is a medical concern? (i.e. painful acne, rosacea, eczema, psoriasis, a rash)

If you answer 'yes' or 'unsure', you should speak to your GP.
Your GP may be able to make an initial diagnosis, prescribe medication and/or refer you on to someone who will be able to guide you further, such as a dermatologist or dietitian. Once you have spoken to your GP, I believe it is worthwhile to speak with a skin therapist about a well-rounded skincare routine that can work alongside GP (or dermatologist) advice.

If you answer 'no', have you spoken to a skin therapist or aesthetic skin consultant before?

If not, you should speak to a skin consultant.
An expert skin consultant will be able to guide you on what cosmetic, active and cosmeceutical skincare will benefit your skin, if what you're using is right for you and if they believe you need to speak with another part of the skin professional jigsaw puzzle. They will also be able to tell you whether you should speak with a GP, dermatologist, dietitian or other professional.

If yes, do you think your concern could be related to an internal health concern related to diet?

If that might be the case, ask your GP about a referral to a dietitian or nutritional specialist.

Do you feel that a lack of exercise is contributing to your skin health?

If yes, speak to an exercise expert.

A personal trainer, or another exercise expert, is a valuable resource, not because it's impossible to create your own exercise routine, but because they can provide you with a routine that will work for you (ringing any bells? It's our whole philosophy), allowing you to ease in without being put off by a daunting and perhaps scary-sounding workout plan. Exercise is integral to skin health as it promotes circulation, allowing for the nutrients in food to reach our skin sharpish. Exercise can also help to reduce feelings of stress, which, as we've learned in Chapter 3 (page 35), can have a knock-on effect on our skin.

Do you feel that your feelings about your skin don't improve even if your skin improves?

If yes, speak to a mental health professional.

If your ongoing skin struggles have improved with time and treatment, yet you do not feel much better in your own skin, counselling and therapy can help you to improve feelings of self-worth and how you see yourself, and can help you to organise your feelings and understand them better. Improved stress levels may mean that your skin concerns can improve too.

Part Three Skin Takeaways

- You need to have a skincare regime – one that works for *your* skin and suits your needs, wallet and time. This means targeted, hard-working products and less of them on the shelf. The very best approach is an A.M. and P.M. approach, which means you bookend your day with a bit of 'me time'. Who could say no to that?

- In terms of active skincare that delivers results, **serums are your best friend**. Now you know that primary and secondary serums are a good option – one for overall skin health, one for targeted results. It's worth figuring out what you need, and which serums will best deliver it for you.

- You are very aware by now that there is a broad network of people out there who can help with all aspects of skincare – and I hope that's a reassuring thought! The **expert jigsaw** (see page 198) is equipped to deal with every skin concern imaginable, so you never have to go it alone. Know this.

- If you're thinking about seeking professional help and feel confused by where to turn, a skin consultation is one helpful route, but **your GP is a portal to all the other disciplines**. They can assess your particular concerns and offer medical help, or they can refer you on to the correct expert. It's an easy way to get guidance and support.

- If you take one thing away from these chapters, I hope that it's the fact that you deserve to feel good in your own skin and that you can do so much to make that happen.

Personal Action Plan

Here is an example of a Personal Action Plan where you can take note of any advice relevant to your lifestyle and your skin goals – it's your personal tailor-made guide on what to do next.

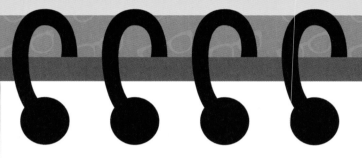

Questions for Personal Action Plan

What do I like about my skin?
(Examples: dewy, plump, few lines, very clear, never dry)

What do I want to improve about my skin?
(Examples: better hydration, less visible lines,
less congestion, glowier, softer, fewer dry patches)

What can I do?
- **A)** internally – nutrition, lifestyle (e.g. cut down on caffeine, eat more antioxidants)
- **B)** topically - (e.g. add antioxidants, exfoliate less, change cleansers)
- **C)** on top - (e.g. wear SPF daily, switch to mineral makeup)

What expert can I talk to about my concerns?

Conclusion

So, we've reached the end of our skinversation – too many nerdisms? Never! – and hopefully you've found that this book has given you the knowledge and the encouragement you need to set off or continue on your multi-disciplinary path to good skin health. Make sure to keep in mind all aspects of caring for your skin, focusing on the essential 360° approach, and think about what you will do differently moving forward. I hope you will consider new ways to think about skin concerns and how your feelings about your skin might affect your mental health. Maybe you will decide to add new steps or ingredients into your routine. Maybe you will read ingredients lists more carefully with all your newly-gained knowledge and you won't be afraid to dig into some reliable research. Or maybe you will have realised that now is the time to seek expert advice. Start with your Personal Action Plan (see page 3 for a reminder), which I know you've been diligently keeping like a good student (right?). You've taken in a lot of information so now you need to figure out what is most relevant and – the most important bit – you need to follow through on that. You are your own skin saviour, you are your own best advocate, you are the defender supreme of your own skindividual health. Own it, hoomans!

And remember it's okay to need help with this, so please do seek out expert assessment and advice, especially if you have an ongoing skin condition that hasn't responded to your efforts to calm it. We would love you to join the Nerd Network, that's a given! You're cordially invited, RSVP expected.

Jennifer Rock

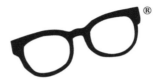

Disclaimer: There are a few hard-set favourite products and brands mentioned, with some newer discoveries included too. Skincare is always evolving so we study the science and evolve with it! At the time of printing, these are the products and brands that we truly rate and recommend on our social platforms and to our loyal Nerd Networkers.

The Skin Nerd
Skincare Community

In case you would like some more information on the Nerd Network, our website, my first book, etc., here is a quick synopsis of all of it and details about how to get in touch with us. Do come say hi to us on our channels – we're a friendly bunch!

Nerd Network Online Skin Consultations – theskinnerd.com/nerdnetwork

The Nerd Network is your first step towards long-term skin health and real results with the guidance of a qualified and experienced skin expert (we call them Nerds and Nerdettes). Once you've booked in, you become a member of the Nerd Network, our skincare guidance community. As a Nerd Network member, you can have a full initial consultation, follow-up consultations and touchpoints with a skin expert Nerd or Nerdette whenever you need. You gain access to exclusive Nerd Network blog posts and videos plus live Q&As and you'll be invited to Nerd Network exclusive events.

Your carefully selected results-driven skincare routine is shipped directly to your door so there's no need to peruse shelves if you don't enjoy browsing or if you don't have time. When you're a member, you can also contact us for skin advice for even the smallest of skin queries. As a Nerd Networker, we support you however we can to help you feel more skin confident. You can also have an online skin consultation with our nerdie GP with a special interest in dermatology, Dr Olga, if recommended by your Nerd or Nerdette.

Our approach is based on the famous 360° philosophy: skincare that is internal (nutrition and wellbeing), on the outside (topical skincare) and on top (SPF and makeup). We listen and try to skinvestigate what could be the root of your concerns, and our robust consultation form, completed by our members prior to their initial consultation, allows us to study aspects of your skin before we even speak with you for the first time. We are accountable for your skin, like a personal trainer, and we can work towards your budget – additionally, we aren't biased towards our own brand as we stock more than 30 other brands with more curated offerings being added all the time.

There is a variety of options to suit you best: Teen Nerd Network, Pregnancy Nerd Network, Bridal Nerd Network and, of course, the original Nerd Network. All of them work towards your specific goals, the difference is how we go about it. We also have an OTI-certified (Oncology Training International) Nerd who can consult with those going through cancer treatment and those who are in remission.

All of our one-to-one video consultations are carried out online, wherever you feel most comfortable, anywhere on the planet.

Not to sound twee in any way, but Nerd Network isn't just skin support … It's a bit of soul support, with real qualified consultants to help you find your way and maintain skin health.

Skingredients: available from skingredients.com and selected pharmacies, salons, clinics and department stores across Ireland

Skingredients is an active skincare range created to mirror the nutrients your skin needs, with vitamins, fats, fruit, veg and botanical extracts.

The nerdie store – theskinnerd.com

Alongside the Nerd Network, we stock more than 30 brands on our online store – everything from supplements, to pre-serums, exfoliating treatments, lip balm and makeup. You name it. The store began as a place to offer a selection of our favourite cosmetic and active skincare products, skincare that you may find difficult to find, or at least difficult to find all in one place.

It's your one-stop shop, making it easy for you to have a full, well-rounded skincare routine delivered straight to your door, and speedily too. We ship across the entire globe so that Ireland can experience some of the best of the world's skincare, and the world can experience some of the best of Ireland's skincare.

Cleanse Off Mitt: available at cleanseoffmitt.com and selected pharmacies, salons, clinics and department stores across Ireland

The COM is a microfibre, reusable pre-cleansing and cleansing tool that removes makeup with just water. It's created for all skins, all ages and all genders, and is ideal as an alternative to wipes or micellar water and cotton pads.

The Skin Nerd: Your Straight-Talking Guide to Feeding, Protecting & Respecting Your Skin

If you have not read the first book, *The Skin Nerd*, let me explain: it is a wide-ranging introduction to skincare, including explanations of skin anatomy and physiology, the basics of a skincare routine, key ingredients, with plenty of practical information on how to carry out your skincare routine to your best ability. It covers specific skin concerns in great detail and discusses how best to look after your skin, inside, outside and on top. I am grateful for the fact that it was a bestseller, and to this day I receive messages from those who have read it. I love that it has become something that spreads the word about the nerdie community, another avenue of skin education.

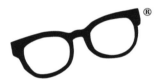

Expert Contributors

I would like to acknowledge and thank the following for their expert and extremely helpful contributions to this book:

Melanie Murphy

www.melaniemurphy.ie

Melanie Murphy is a two-time bestselling author of *Fully Functioning Human (Almost)* and *If Only* and an award-winning online content creator from Dublin. She has over 800,000 followers across her social media platforms, reaching people with her warm personality and her life lessons as well as her views on divisive topics such as sexuality, women's rights, health and relationships.

Holly White

www.holly.ie

Holly White is a broadcaster, journalist and author. Having been vegan for 5 years and having trained extensively with some of the best vegan chefs in the world, she is all about injecting flavour into vegan food while keeping it quick and practical to prepare. She is certified in plant-based nutrition from Cornell University, and her debut cookbook *Vegan-ish* was published in September 2018.

Caroline Foran

www.carolineforan.com

Caroline Foran is a number one bestselling author of two, soon to be three, non-fiction books, *Owning It: Your Bullsh*t-Free Guide To Living With Anxiety*,

The Confidence Kit and, coming January 2021, *NAKED: Ten Truths To Change Your Life*. Outside of writing books, Caroline is known for her hit podcast Owning It: The Anxiety Podcast which has enjoyed over one and a quarter million downloads.

Lydia Sasse

www.instagram.com/yogawithlydia

Yoga has been a life-long pursuit of Lydia's, but to give her a greater understanding of how the body works and why it sometimes doesn't, Lydia has also trained as a Bowen therapist and completed a diploma in physiology and anatomy. She is a qualified Hatha yoga teacher, teacher trainer, women's health yoga therapist and wellness coach and speaker. Lydia has specialised in a lot of the more unique areas of yoga and has a love of yoga for the face and eyes.

Níall Ó Murchú

www.breathewithniall.com

We can transform our lives by simply breathing, using nature and a little bit of cold. That is why Níall Ó Murchú became a herbalist, traditional Irish healer and Wim Hof Method instructor: to help people transform how they feel and think for the better. It has helped him to be a better father, a better husband and a better man.

Dr Alia Ahmed, BSc, DRCOG, MRCP

www.thepsychodermatologist.com

Dr Alia Ahmed is a consultant dermatologist working for Frimley and Barts Health NHS Trusts. She graduated from Barts and the Royal London School of Medicine in 2008 and completed her dermatology training in London, including a research fellowship in psychodermatology, becoming a consultant in 2017. Dr Ahmed also has a BSc in Psychology with Clinical Psychology (University of Kent). In addition to her NHS work, Dr Ahmed is an honorary lecturer in psychodermatology at the University of Hertfordshire.

Orla Walsh

www.orlawalshnutrition.ie
Born in Dublin, Orla is a qualified dietitian and member of the Irish Nutrition and Dietetic Institute (MINDI) and Self Employed Dietitians of Ireland (SEDI). Orla qualified as a dietitian from King's College London, and has since obtained an MA in Physiology, a master's in Clinical Nutrition and a postgraduate diploma in Sports and Exercise Nutrition.

Dr Callaghan Condon, MB, Bch, BAO, DTM, MRCPI, MD

Dr Cal Condon is a consultant in medical and surgical dermatology at UPMC Kildare Hospital and the Blackrock Clinic. Having studied general medicine in Dublin for 3 years, Cal commenced as registrar at the South Infirmary Hospital in Cork and from there became a clinical and research Fellow at the University of Pittsburgh and Pittsburgh Cancer Institute. His work in Pittsburgh led to his being awarded a medical doctorate from UCD and the Jacob Medal in Dermatology by the Irish Association of Dermatologists.

Mr Kambiz Golchin, MMED SCI, FRCS (ORL-HNS)

www.kambizgolchin.com
Mr Kambiz Golchin is an assistant clinical professor and an ENT consultant & facial plastic surgeon whose pioneering techniques have gained international acclaim. He is the founder of Beacon Face & Dermatology on the Beacon Medical Campus and offers pioneering skin rejuvenating treatments at Dr Rakus's Knightsbridge Clinic, London. He has operating facilities in top hospitals in Dublin and London.

Dr Olga O'Driscoll, MB, BCh, BAO, ICGP, PGDip AM (Aesthetic Medicine)

www.athenrysurgery.ie / www.medicalaesthetics.ie

Dr Olga O'Driscoll is a medical graduate of NUI Galway, and of the Irish College of General Practitioners. She has worked in various fields of hospital medicine including paediatrics, obstetrics, emergency medicine, psychiatry, and general internal medicine. Through her work as a GP she developed a keen interest in women's health and dermatology and went on to complete a Postgraduate Diploma in Aesthetic Medicine through Queen Mary University, London.

Oonagh O'Hagan

www.meaghers.ie

Oonagh O'Hagan is a qualified pharmacist and the owner and managing director of the Meaghers Pharmacy Group, a group of nine physical pharmacies in Dublin and the thriving online store meaghers.ie, serving customers all over the world. Keen to help shape and reposition the role of the pharmacist in the Irish healthcare system, Oonagh has held positions in the Pharmaceutical Society of Ireland and also sits on the strategic board in the School of Pharmacy, Trinity College Dublin.

Jeanne Brophy

www.jeannebrophy.com

An award-winning facialist, Jeanne Brophy has a passion for delivering optimum skin health. Jeanne's approach is results driven while respecting the delicate balance the skin needs to thrive. Her bespoke treatments marry the most up-to-date clinical treatments with targeted massage and active ingredients. Alongside her facial work at the Jeanne Brophy Skin Clinic, Jeanne is also a respected educator teaching advanced skin analysis and treatments.

Karl Henry, BSc, AABS, ACE

www.karlhenry.ie

Karl Henry is one of Ireland's most recognised and leading personal trainers. Renowned as personal trainer to the stars, Karl is responsible for creating some of the most famous physiques in fashion, music, politics and the corporate world. He is well known for his role as the leading fitness expert on RTÉ One's *Operation Transformation* since it began twelve years ago. In 2018, Karl released his fifth book called *Karl Henry's Healthy Living Handbook*. He is the host of The Real Health Podcast with Karl Henry.

Margaret O'Rourke Doherty

www.imageskillnet.ie / www.habic.ie

Margaret O'Rourke Doherty has been immersed in the hair and beauty industry for two decades. She has earned a CIDESCO Diploma in Beauty and Spa Management in addition to postgraduate diplomas in Management, Leadership, and Strategy & Innovation, and completed her MBA in 2019. She was one of the founding members of the Hair and Beauty Industry Confederation (HABIC) and the founder of IMAGE Skillnet, a dedicated network for supporting the Irish beauty and hair sector with subsidised, tailored training.

Dr Clíodhna O'Donovan

instagram.com/drcliodhnaodonovan

Senior counselling psychologist, C. Psychol., PsSI (Chartered Psychologist of the Psychological Society of Ireland, PSI)

Dr Clíodhna O'Donovan is a senior psychologist with a doctorate in Counselling Psychology obtained at Trinity College Dublin. Dr O'Donovan has worked across a wide range of services with children and adults and has specialised in mental health, intellectual disability, and neuropsychological assessments. She also provides consultancy to *Stellar* magazine on feature articles with psychological underpinnings, such as an exploration of perfectionism and the influence of social media on self-esteem.

Dr Katherine Mulrooney, MB BCh BAO, MSc. Clinical Dermatology

www.drmulrooney.com

Dr Katherine Mulrooney specialises exclusively in the treatment of ageing skin. After studying medicine at NUI Galway, she completed a master's degree in Clinical Dermatology at the renowned St John's Institute of Dermatology at St Thomas' Hospital in London and thereafter has gained more than 15 years' experience exclusively in cosmetic dermatology. She is co-founder of The Dr Mulrooney Clinic and the co-owner and medical director of SEAVITE Skincare.

Millie Kendall, MBE

www.britishbeautycouncil.com

During her career as a brand creator, Millie Kendall has been essential to the success of well-known brands including Shu Uemura, Aveda, Tweezerman, L'Occitane and Ruby & Millie. In 1998, Millie Kendall and Ruby Hammer launched Ruby & Millie, and in 2007, both Ruby and Millie were awarded an MBE for services to the cosmetic industry. In 2018, with Anna-Marie Solowij and Kate Shapland, Millie Kendall founded the British Beauty Council, a non-profit organisation that aims to support a successful, innovative, and inclusive British beauty industry.

Acknowledgements

Hachette Ireland have been, again, a constant support throughout this process. Thank you for always acting to translate my desires and ideas for this book into what the reader would want. The timeline was tight as ever, and your allowing me to squeeze every last nerdie word in is very much appreciated. Lucy Bennett of Team Nerd was the rock in-house to ensure all was in line with our high expectations, and never ceases to amaze me with her relentless enthusiasm for all things written word, Nerd style.

To all of the contributors, of which there are many, I respect you endlessly and yearn to learn from you both personally and professionally. Thank you for dedicating your time to provide advice to our readers. It gives me great hope for the sector to see so many professionals advocate for a multi-disciplinary approach. I welcome the future that professionals like the contributors will bring.

I'd be remiss if I failed to mention my friends and family, always at the other end of the phone for support, to motivate me or simply to listen, in particular Jill and Joan, and Sinead, Sharon and Mr Price, AKA my three musketeers. Claire, Cat, Kate, Ellen and Orna will always have a girl's back, from bottle green uniforms to white nerdie lab coats and all that has been in between.

To Paul, the man with a plan – as always, your attention to detail and advice has been a guiding light through trying times. And to my entire team for supporting thousands of clients, each receiving the love and attention they deserve – this team are the true operation and nerdie force.

To each and every hooman who has supported the .com, Skingredients or who is a Nerd Network member, to all who email, DM, live-chat with us, and believe in and echo our ethos and philosophies – thank you. I will never, ever take this for granted. It is an honour to be able to assist you via the power of education; thank you for pushing me to want to learn so that I can then relay it all back – and here's hoping for many, many more years of same.

Also to all stockists, my agent Amy, my distributor and to my special group of mentors whom I name Pearl – I would not be the hooman I am without your undivided support, attention and space to learn and grow.

There are so many to acknowledge both personally and professionally but I would hope I say it to them regularly in hooman too. Life is fast-paced and, delicious indeed as that is, we need to stop to acknowledge many hoomans as time goes by.

'Don't wait for big moments' is my philosophy; see and thank and appreciate as you go. So thank you to you, the reader – your dedicated support and relentless yearning to learn is the reason I get to do what I do daily. Thank you.